Manual of Ambulatory General Surgery

Springer
*London
Berlin
Heidelberg
New York
Barcelona
Hong Kong
Milan
Paris
Santa Clara
Singapore
Tokyo*

Shukri K. Shami and Delilah A. Hassanally

Manual of Ambulatory General Surgery

A Step-by-Step Guide to Minor and Intermediate Surgery

Foreword by B.F. Ribeiro

Illustrations by Caroline Munklinde

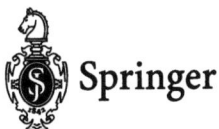
Springer

Shukri K. Shami, MS, FRCS
Consultant General and Vascular Surgeon, Surgical Tutor, Oldchurch Hospital, Havering Hospitals NHS Trust, Waterloo Road, Romford, Essex. RM7 0BE.

Delilah A. Hassanally, BSc, MBBS, FRCS
Specialist Registrar in Surgery, North Thames (East) Rotation, London.

ISBN-13:978-1-4471-1187-0

British Library Cataloguing in Publication Data
Shami, Shukri K.
  Manual of ambulatory general surgery
  1.Ambulatory surgery – Handbooks, manuals, etc.   2.Surgical
  clinics – Handbooks, manuals, etc.
  I.Title II.Hassanally, Delilah A.
  617'.024
  ISBN-13:978-1-4471-1187-0

Library of Congress Cataloging-in-Publication Data
Shami, Shukri K. 1952–
    Manual of ambulatory surgery / Shukri K. Shami and Delilah A. Hassanally.
      p.   cm.
   ISBN-13:978-1-4471-1187-0   e-ISBN-13:978-1-4471-0723-1
   DOI: 10.1007/978-1-4471-0723-1

    1. Ambulatory surgery Handbooks, manuals, etc.   I. Hassanally, Delilah A., 1963–   . II. Title.
    [DNLM: 1. Ambulatory Surgical Procedures Handbooks.   WO 39 S528m 1999]
  RD110.S53   1999
  617'.024—dc21
  DNLM/DLC
  for Library of Congress   99-17030

Apart from any fair dealing for the purposes of research or private study, or criticism or review, as permitted under the Copyright, Designs and Patents Act 1988, this publication may only be reproduced, stored or transmitted, in any form or by any means, with the prior permission in writing of the publishers, or in the case of reprographic reproduction in accordance with the terms of licences issued by the Copyright Licensing Agency. Enquiries concerning reproduction outside those terms should be sent to the publishers.

© Springer-Verlag London Limited 2000
Softcover reprint of the hardcover 1st edition 2000

The use of registered names, trademarks, etc. in this publication does not imply, even in the absence of a specific statement, that such names are exempt from the relevant laws and regulations and therefore free for general use.

Product liability: The publisher can give no guarantee for information about drug dosage and application thereof contained in this book. In every individual case the respective user must check its accuracy by consulting other pharmaceutical literature.

Typeset by Florence Production Limited, Stoodleigh, Devon, England

28/3830-543210 Printed on acid-free paper SPIN 10508602

We would like to dedicate this book to our parents

S.K. Shami
D.A. Hassanally

Foreword

It is rare to find a text book of surgery specifically written for GPs and SHOs.

This is a refreshing book which sets out safe methods of practice and defines situations in which common surgical procedures can be undertaken. The emphasis is on a clear diagnosis, and safe execution of the surgical procedure.

The authors have clearly identified the level of surgical expertise and knowledge required to undertake these procedures, and offer useful tips as to how these can be performed. Increasingly SHOs enter surgical practice without the rigour of the primary FRCS. They need guidance and assistance to explain operative procedures, and these are provided through clear text and diagrams.

The ambulatory surgery described in this book is based on practice in the United Kingdom, where SHOs perform surgery under supervision. The principles outlined in this book are common to all practitioners, and they will be equally helpful to doctors working outside the United Kingdom.

B.F. Ribeiro, FRCS
Consultant Surgeon, Basildon Hospital, Nether Mayne,
Basildon, Essex SS16 5NL
President of the Association of Surgeons of Great Britain and Ireland
Member of the Council of the Royal College of Surgeons of England

Contents

Introduction		xv
1	**General Principles**	1
	1.1 Introduction	1
	1.2 Scrubbing and Gowning	1
	1.3 Skin Preparation and Draping	3
	1.4 Antibiotic Prophylaxis	3
	1.4.1 Principles	3
	1.4.2 Types of Antibiotics, Dosages and Routes of Administration	5
	1.4.3 Timing of Prophylactic Antibiotics	5
	1.5 Protection against HIV and Hepatitis	5
	1.6 Accidental Contamination	6
	1.6.1 Contamination of the Operation Field	6
	1.6.2 Contamination of a Member of the Operating Team	6
	1.7 Patient Consent and Medico-legal Aspects	6
	1.7.1 Consent	7
	1.7.2 Operation Record	7
	1.7.3 Medical Notes	8
2	**Instruments, Sutures and Diathermy**	9
	2.1 Introduction	9
	2.2 Instrumentation	9
	2.2.1 Scalpels	9
	2.2.2 Forceps	10
	2.2.3 Needle Holders	10
	2.2.4 Retractors	10
	2.2.5 Curettes	12
	2.2.6 Infiltration Needles	12
	2.2.7 Tourniquets	12
	2.3 Sutures	12
	2.3.1 Principles	12

		2.3.2	Materials	13
		2.3.3	Technique	13
		2.3.4	Needles	15
		2.3.5	Knots	17
		2.3.6	Clips and Staples	18
		2.3.7	Removal of Sutures and Clips	18
	2.4	Diathermy		19
		2.4.1	Monopolar (unipolar)	19
		2.4.2	Bipolar	20
3	**Anaesthetics**			21
	3.1	Introduction		21
	3.2	Types of Local Anaesthetics		21
		3.2.1	Short-acting Local Anaesthetics	21
		3.2.2	Long-acting Local Anaesthetics	22
		3.2.3	Mixtures	22
		3.2.4	Precautions	22
	3.3	Local Infiltration		23
	3.4	Ring Block		24
	3.5	Nerve Block		25
4	**Vascular Access**			27
	4.1	Introduction		27
	4.2	Venous Cutdown		27
	4.3	Central Lines		28
		4.3.1	Subclavian Vein Access	29
		4.3.2	Internal Jugular Vein Access	31
	4.4	Total Parenteral Nutrition and Tunnelled Venous Lines		32
5	**Lesions of the Skin and Subcutaneous Tissue**			35
	5.1	Introduction		35
	5.2	Lacerations		35
		5.2.1	Suturing Lacerations	35
		5.2.2	Other Methods of Closing Skin Lacerations	36
		5.2.3	Special Cases	37
	5.3	Skin Tag and Papilloma		37
	5.4	Sebaceous Cyst		38
	5.5	Dermoid Cyst		39
	5.6	Lipoma		40

	5.7	Pigmented Naevus	41
	5.8	Keloid Scar	42
	5.9	Abscess	43
	5.10	Skin Cancers	44
		5.10.1 Basal Cell Carcinoma	44
		5.10.2 Squamous Cell Carcinoma	45
		5.10.3 Malignant Melanoma	45
	5.11	Pinch Skin Graft	47
	5.12	Warts and Verrucas	48
	5.13	Skin Biopsy	49
	5.14	Other Lesions	50
		5.14.1 Solar Keratosis	50
		5.14.2 Seborrheic Wart	50
		5.14.3 Bowen's Disease	50
		5.14.4 Miscellaneous Skin Lesions	50
6	**Varicose Veins**	51
	6.1	Introduction	51
	6.2	Indications for Surgery	51
	6.3	Investigations	51
	6.4	Treatment Rationale	52
		6.4.1 Sapheno-femoral Junction Incompetence with Long Saphenous Varices	52
		6.4.2 Sapheno-popliteal Junction Incompetence with Short Saphenous Varices	52
		6.4.3 Combined Sapheno-femoral and Sapheno-popliteal Junction Incompetence with Long and Short Saphenous Varices	53
		6.4.4 Varicosities with no Junction Incompetence	53
		6.4.5 Calf Perforator Incompetence	53
	6.5	Recurrent Varicose Veins	53
	6.6	Sclerotherapy	53
	6.7	Junction Ligation	56
		6.7.1 Sapheno-femoral Junction	56
		6.7.2 Sapheno-popliteal Junction	59
	6.8	Stripping	61
		6.8.1 Conventional Stripping	61
		6.8.2 Inversion stripping	64
	6.9	Avulsion of Varicosities (Phlebectomies)	65
	6.10	Post-operative Care	65

7 Hernia Repair ... 69
- 7.1 Introduction ... 69
- 7.2 Inguinal Hernia ... 69
- 7.3 Femoral Hernia ... 76
- 7.4 Para-umbilical Hernia ... 77
- 7.5 Other Herniae ... 79

8 Anal Procedures ... 81
- 8.1 Introduction ... 81
- 8.2 Investigative Procedures ... 81
  - 8.2.1 Proctoscopy ... 81
  - 8.2.2 Rigid Sigmoidoscopy ... 82
  - 8.2.3 Flexible Sigmoidoscopy ... 83
- 8.3 Examination under Anaesthesia (EUA) ... 84
- 8.4 Haemorrhoids ... 85
  - 8.4.1 Injection of Haemorrhoids ... 85
  - 8.4.2 Banding of Haemorrhoids ... 86
- 8.5 Skin Tags ... 87
- 8.6 Anal Fissure ... 88
  - 8.6.1 Anal Stretch ... 89
  - 8.6.2 Lateral (Internal) Sphincterotomy ... 90
- 8.7 Fistula-in-Ano ... 92
- 8.8 Anal Warts ... 95

9 Miscellaneous ... 99
- 9.1 Ganglion ... 99
- 9.2 Procedures on Nails ... 100
  - 9.2.1 Paronychia ... 100
  - 9.2.2 Subungual Haematoma ... 101
  - 9.2.3 Simple Avulsion of Nail ... 102
  - 9.2.4 Lateral Wedge Excision ... 102
  - 9.2.5 Zadek's Operation ... 104
- 9.3 Muscle Biopsy ... 105
- 9.4 Temporal Artery Biopsy ... 107
- 9.5 Amputation of a Toe ... 108
- 9.6 Catheterisation ... 110
  - 9.6.1 Urethral Catheterisation ... 110
  - 9.6.2 Suprapubic Catheterisation ... 116
- 9.7 Circumcision ... 116

	9.7.1 Conventional Technique	117
	9.7.2 Plastibell Technique	120
9.8	Vasectomy	120

Appendices

Appendix A	Scrub and Operative Field Preparation Solutions	123
Appendix B	Dosages of Popular Local Anaesthetics, Sedatives and Analgesics used in Local Anaesthetic Operations	125
Appendix C	Prophylactic Antibiotic Regimens and Dosages	127
Appendix D	Consent Forms	129
Appendix E	Medical Defence Organisations in the UK	131

Index 133

Introduction

This book aims to give a step-by-step guide to general surgical operations performed as day-case procedures. Most of the operations described can be performed under local anaesthetic; however, some require general anaesthesia. We have concentrated on operations and procedures that would be undertaken in a general surgical practice.

The book is aimed mainly at two groups of people: (1) junior doctors, particularly pre-registration house surgeons (PRHO) and senior house officers (SHO), who may undertake such procedures, and (2) general practitioners who may wish to undertake minor and intermediate surgery. It may also be of interest to medical students and nurses.

It is not our intention for this book to be a reference book on surgery, nor an exhaustive textbook of operative surgery. The aim is to provide a practical guide and an *aide-mémoire* for persons not totally familiar with the procedures described, enabling them to carry out the procedures safely.

The chapters on varicose vein surgery and hernia repair are directed particularly at SHOs. We do not feel that these operations are suitable for GPs to do as we feel that they should be done in a hospital setting. They are also too complex to be undertaken by PRHOs.

The importance of getting proper supervised training in the techniques of surgery cannot be overstressed, and this book in no way replaces that. We do not recommend for anyone to undertake any of the procedures described without adequate training first.

We are indebted to Mr. S. Sarin, Consultant Surgeon, Watford General Hospital, Mr. T. Cheatle, Consultant Surgeon, Norfolk & Norwich Hospital and Mr. S. Ahmed, Specialist Registrar in Surgery, Oldchurch Hospital, for reviewing the manuscript and for their helpful suggestions. We are also indebted to Theatre 4 staff in Oldchurch Hospital (particularly Joan, Carol, Terri and Deena), medical photography at Oldchurch Hospital and Ms Jane Armstrong at Basildon Hospital for their help.

We hope you find this book helpful, and that it helps you perform the operations described in a safe and competent manner.

S. K. Shami and D. A. Hassanally

1 General Principles

1.1 Introduction

This chapter concentrates on the topics that are relevant to every operation. These include protecting the patient against endogenous and exogenous infections during surgery, protecting the surgeon against infections that may be acquired from the patient, and ensuring that the operation is done in a "legal" and defensible manner. All the procedures described in this manual should be done in a specially designed operating theatre using sterile technique.

1.2 Scrubbing and Gowning

"Greens" (operating room attire – head cover, mask, operating suit, theatre shoes or shoe covers) should be worn in an operation suite. The purpose of this is to prevent the spread of micro-organisms to the patient from the operating team by providing an effective barrier. "Greens" should not be worn outside the operation suite, and masks should be changed between cases.

"Scrubbing" consists of cleaning the hands and forearms (up to the elbows) using an antiseptic solution prior to "gowning". The purpose of this is to remove as many micro-organisms from the skin as possible mechanically as well as a result of the antiseptic solution. Scrubbing is recommended for a period of three minutes. Scrubbing that is too vigorous, especially with a brush, may cause abrasions and should be avoided. Scrubbing consists of cleaning the fingers (all sides), the nails, the rest of the hand and the forearm. At least three applications of the antiseptic is needed. During rinsing, it is important to keep the hands above the level of the elbows so that the water and antiseptic drain away from the hand rather than carry potentially dirty fluid from the elbow area to the hands.

Popular scrubbing solutions include povidone-iodine and chlorhexidine. After scrubbing you should clasp your hands together at a level higher than the elbows and walk to the gowning area. A sterile gown, sterile disposable towels, and a pair of sterile gloves, should have been placed for you.

- Dry each hand using the sterile towels and discard them without touching anything unsterile. Start by drying the hand, then go up the forearm up to the elbow.
- Take the gown and unfold it.
- Hold it so that you can see where to place your arms.
- Insert each arm but do not push your hand out beyond the wrist cuff.

2 Manual of Ambulatory General Surgery

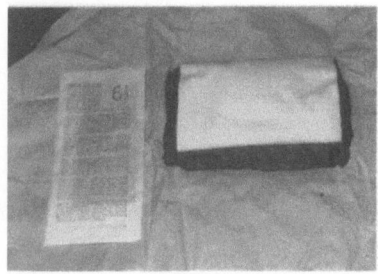

1 Sterile gown, towel and a pair of gloves laid out in a sterile manner

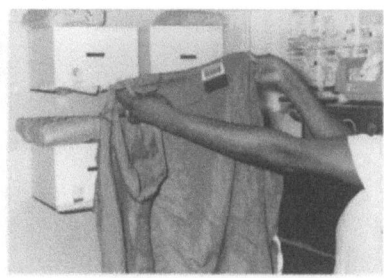

2 After scrubbing put on the gown (only by touching the inside). Do not push hands through the sleeves of the gown

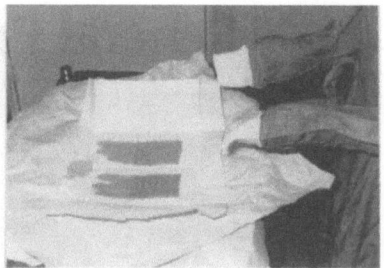

3 Unfold the packet containing the sterile gloves

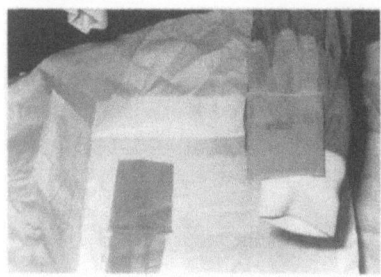

4 Rest the appropriate glove of one hand on the hand as shown. Orient the glove so that the thumb of the glove is opposed to the thumb of the hand with the fingers of the glove pointing up the arm. Push the tips of the fingers (still covered by the sleeve of the gown) through the opening in the glove to grasp the glove

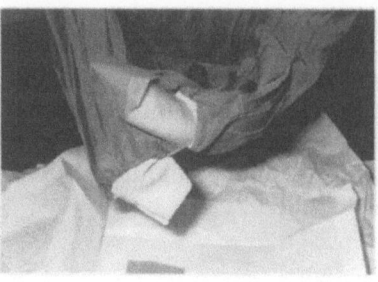

5 Use the other hand to unfold the wrist of the glove onto the first hand

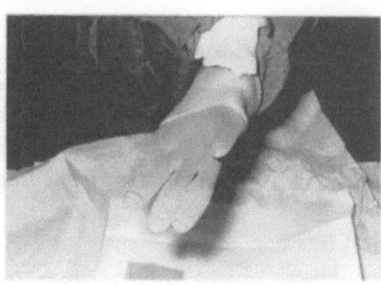

6 With the other hand, grasp the wrist of the glove and the sleeve of the gown underneath it and pull proximally to slide the hand into the glove

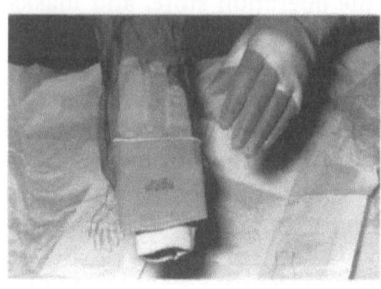

7–9 Repeat steps 4–6 above for the other hand

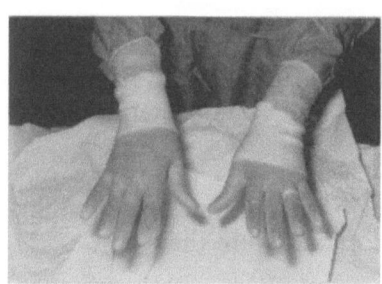

10 You are now ready for action!

Figure 1.1. Putting on gloves

- Get an assistant to tie the back of the gown.
- Put on the sterile gloves as shown in Figure 1.1.

1.3 Skin Preparation and Draping

Before operating on a patient, the skin of the area of operation must be prepared by disinfecting it and draping it with sterile towels. The aim is to try and remove as many micro-organisms as possible. It is preferable to shave the area of any hair first (this should be done as close to the start of the operation as practical in order to avoid infection of cuts or abrasions caused by shaving – a clipper or depilating agent may avoid this problem). Shaving the skin will avoid hair getting into the wound, as well as make it easier to apply a sticky adhesive dressing to cover the wound after the operation. The skin then needs to be cleaned with an antiseptic solution such as povidone-iodine (alcoholic or aqueous) or chlorhexidine solution. Alcoholic solutions should not be applied on mucous membranes.

- Prepare the area using a sponge or swab on a holder soaked in the antiseptic solution.
- If a limb is being prepared, have an assistant elevate the limb; start distally and work proximally.
- Try and ensure that the whole area and a reasonable area beyond the area of operation is prepared.
- Do this again using a second "sponge on a stick".
- If a limb is being prepared, ask a "sterile" assistant to place a sterile towel below the limb and then have the limb lowered onto the towel.
- Now cover the perimeter of the operation field with sterile towels and secure them to each other using towel clips or sterile adhesive strips.
- Only the prepared area should be visible.
- The operative "field" is now ready.

1.4 Antibiotic Prophylaxis

1.4.1 Principles

Antibiotic prophylaxis is used when there is a significant risk of wound infection that can be reduced by giving pre- or per-operative **prophylactic** antibiotics (this must not be confused with antibiotic treatment for established infection). In general, operations can be divided into four categories: clean, potentially contaminated (clean-contaminated), contaminated and dirty. Definitions and examples of each of these categories are shown in Table 1.1.

Table 1.2 below shows the approximate wound infection rate with and without prophylactic antibiotics for each of those categories.

In clean operations, a hundred patients would need to be given prophylactic antibiotics in order to save only one from a wound infection. Since giving antibiotics carries a small risk, with such minimal benefits it is considered inappropriate to give

Table 1.1. Categorization of operations

Category	Definition	Examples
Clean	An operation through structures that are not infected and are sterile	• Excision of lipoma • Excision of breast lump
Potentially contaminated (clean-contaminated)	An operation through structures that are not infected and are **normally** sterile, but may contain organisms under certain circumstances	• Procedures on the urinary bladder • Gall bladder operations
Contaminated	An operation through structures that always contain organisms	• Operations on the mouth, vagina, anus • Operations on the large bowel including the appendix
Dirty	An operation through infected tissue	• Incision and drainage of an abscess

prophylactic antibiotics in these patients except in special circumstances (see below). In patients with dirty wounds, the wound is usually left open to drain, and most of these patients will already be on antibiotics for treatment purposes. Therefore prophylactic antibiotics in this group are also not appropriate. It can thus be appreciated that only patients undergoing "potentially contaminated" and "contaminated" operations benefit from prophylactic antibiotics. However, there are special circumstances when prophylactic antibiotics should **always** be used whichever type of operation is being undertaken. These include

- immuno-compromised patients (including patients on immuno-suppressants)
- patients on steroids
- patients with artificial material previously implanted (for example heart valves)
- patients with heart murmurs due to valvular disease
- operations where a foreign material is to be implanted (for example a metal, vascular or other type of prosthesis).

Table 1.2. Approximate wound infection rates for the four categories of operation

Category	Wound infection rate **without** prophylactic antibiotics (%)	Wound infection rate **with** prophylactic antibiotics (%)
Clean	2	1
Potentially contaminated (clean-contaminated)	15	5
Contaminated	40	15
Dirty	100	100

1.4.2 Types of Antibiotics, Dosages and Routes of Administration

Two schools of thought exist regarding which antibiotics to use for prophylaxis. One school suggests targeting the antibiotic against the organisms likely to cause the problem, while the other school suggests the use of broad-spectrum antibiotics to cover the majority of organisms. In general we favour the latter, except for urological procedures, where we would recommend the use of Gentamicin. For all other procedures a broad-spectrum antibiotic such as a cephalosporin (i.e. Cefuroxime) is sufficient. If bowel surgery is being undertaken then an antibacteroides agent (such as Metronidazole) should be added.

The dosage of antibiotic used is dependent on the patient age and weight, but for prophylaxis, usually a single large dose is used (for example 1.5 g Cefuroxime and 500 mg Metronidazole for bowel surgery in an average 70 kg patient).

The usual route of administration of prophylactic antibiotics is the intravenous route. This is in order to achieve a high tissue concentration of the antibiotic during surgery.

1.4.3 Timing of Prophylactic Antibiotics

For prophylactic antibiotics to prevent wound infection, it is important that the tissue levels of the antibiotic are high during potential contamination of the tissues. As contamination usually only occurs during the procedure and perhaps for a short time afterwards, it is essential that the prophylactic antibiotic is given in a high dose just before the procedure starts. This is why the intravenous route is usually used. If the procedure is prolonged (greater than 4 hours) then a second intra-operative dose is needed. In general, most surgeons also give two post-operative doses (6 and 12 hours after the operation). However, most studies show that this is not needed and that a single pre-operative dose is sufficient.

1.5 Protection against HIV and Hepatitis

If it is suspected that a patient to be operated on is suffering from a serious contagious disease, then certain precautions need to be taken. These include

- ensuring that the patient is placed at the end of the operating list
- ensuring that all unnecessary items are removed from the operating theatre during the procedure
- ensuring that the operating theatre is thoroughly disinfected afterwards
- ensuring that only necessary personnel are allowed into theatre during the procedure
- using only disposable gowns and wearing overshoes; these should be discarded after the procedure
- using visors to protect the eyes from contamination
- ensuring that the operating team wears two pairs of gloves; some manufacturers produce special "double gloves" of different colours so that it is obvious if the outer glove has been breached (you are able to see the colour of the inner glove through the defect)
- using only special "blunt" needles during the procedure

- ensuring that sharp instruments are not passed from one person to the other directly but placed in a receiver such as a kidney dish, which is then passed across
- performing the operation with utmost care to avoid inadvertent contamination.

1.6 Accidental Contamination

1.6.1 Contamination of the Operation Field

Contamination of the operating field can occur inadvertently by several ways, including:

- a "non-sterile" person touching the sterile draping – if this occurs, then further sterile draping is placed over the contaminated ones
- a "sterile" glove or gown touching a non-sterile surface – then the gloves or gown need to be changed in a sterile manner
- a non-sterile object or contaminant getting into the wound (this can be endogenous, for example if the bowel is inadvertently breached during the operation) – then the operation wound needs to be washed using generous quantities of warm sterile normal saline. A broad-spectrum antibiotic (such as tetracycline) or an antiseptic (such as povidone-iodine) is added to the saline solution by some surgeons. However, this probably does not increase the efficacy of the washout. A prophylactic dose of antibiotics must also be given intravenously if this has not already been done (see Section 1.4.1).

1.6.2 Contamination of a Member of the Operating Team

Potential contamination of one of the operating team can occur if tissue fluid, including blood from the patient, is splashed into the eyes or mucous membranes. More seriously, it can result from a needle-stick injury. In these cases the procedure recommended by the occupational health policy of the institution needs to be carefully followed. This will usually include the following, which need to be done immediately:

- mechanical cleansing of the contaminated area using copious quantities of antiseptic solutions such as povidone-iodine and water (only sterile saline or eye-wash in the case of contamination of the eyes)
- blood is withdrawn from the patient and the potentially contaminated person for testing for HIV and Hepatitis (consent to do this needs to be obtained from the patient)
- an "incident" report is completed
- the potentially contaminated person should report to the occupational health department as soon as possible.

1.7 Patient Consent and Medico-legal Aspects

Only persons with malpractice insurance (medical indemnity) should carry out procedures or operations on patients. In the United Kingdom, currently, for National Health

Service (NHS) patients, doctors are covered by the NHS hospital they practise in. However, this does not cover private practice. Appendix E gives the contact addresses of organisations that provide such cover. Doctors should also ensure that they are immunised against the Hepatitis B virus. In the United Kingdom, doctors need to be registered with the General Medical Council (GMC) before they can practise.

1.7.1 Consent

Consent must be obtained before any operation is undertaken. It is also good practice to obtain consent before any invasive procedure is undertaken. Appendix D shows two typical consent forms.

You should ensure that the consent is an "informed consent"; in other words, that the procedure and risks are explained to the patient in a way that the patient can understand. We recommend that the consent form should be written in "everyday" language and devoid of medical jargon so as to ensure that patients understand the procedure proposed. Usually any serious complications and those that occur with a frequency of 1 per cent or more should be mentioned. Ideally the person undertaking the procedure should obtain the consent of the patient. Alternatively, a person capable of performing, or is fully familiar with, the planned procedure should obtain the consent.

If the patient is under age (less than 16 years old in the UK) and is deemed unable to make an informed choice, then consent needs to be obtained from a parent or legal guardian. If a patient is mentally incapacitated no one can give or withhold consent to treatment. Provided the patient complies, you may proceed with the treatment. It is good practice to ensure that another competent clinician agrees with the treatment beforehand. It may also be appropriate to inform the next of kin (while having regard to patient confidentiality). Any deviation from the above will put you at risk. For further information, please read the GMC publication entitled: Seeking the patients' consent: the ethical considerations.

1.7.2 Operation Record

Every time a procedure or operation is performed, an "operation note" should be written. This should be clear and legible and should include:

- date and preferably time of operation
- name of surgeon and assistant(s)
- name of anaesthetist (if any)
- any local anaesthetic or other medication used by the surgeon
- tourniquet time if applicable (see Section 2.2.7)
- name of the operation
- indication or justification for the operation
- incision used
- findings: detail all your findings at the operation
- procedure: write down exactly what took place during the operation including any difficulties encountered and any complications
- closure: write down how the wound was closed and the types of sutures used; it is also desirable to include the type of dressing applied
- document that the "swab and instrument count" was correct

- post-operative instructions regarding care of the wound, observations needed post-operatively and instruction for removal of sutures (if any).

1.7.3 Medical Notes

As well as operation notes, it is important to make sure that up-to-date medical notes are written each time a patient is seen, either before or after an operation. The notes should detail exactly where (outpatients, ward, etc.) and when (date and time) the patient was seen, as well as what was done and what the outcome was. It is also important to document that a history and examination (clerking) took place before the operation, ensuring that the patient was fit enough to undergo the operation and that the operation was indicated.

2. Instruments, Sutures and Diathermy

2.1 Introduction

Correct equipment and instruments are essential to perform surgery successfully. This chapter describes the basic instruments needed to perform day-case surgery with instruction on their correct handling.

Information on suture materials is included to enable you to make the correct choices for your operations.

2.2 Instrumentation

2.2.1 Scalpels

The scalpel is used to make clean neat incisions into the skin and can be used for further dissection. There are disposable scalpels with different blades, or stainless steel non-disposable handles with interchangeable blades.

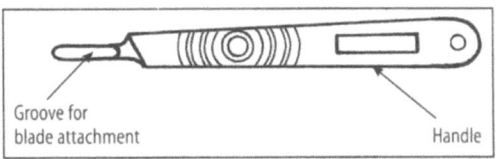

Figure 2.1. Scalpel handle

There are two types of handles: no. 3 and no. 4, which differ simply in the size of the groove for attachment of the blade.

No. 3 handle is used for the smaller blades i.e. 11, 15.
No. 4 handle is used for larger blades i.e. 20, 22.

- No. 10 – this is the usual blade to use for moderate-sized incisions into the skin
- No. 11 – this is a sharp pointed blade used to make "stab" incisions, e.g. for varicose vein avulsion
- No. 15 – this blade is used for small precise incisions. e.g. excision of skin lesions

- No. 20 – this blade is used for larger incisions
- No. 22 – this is a very large blade and is used for very large incisions.

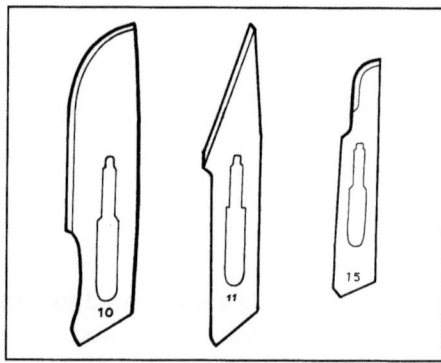

Figure 2.2. Various blades: 10, 11 and 15

The blade is fitted onto one end of the handle by sliding it along a groove. Care should be taken in handling. It is best to use arterial forceps to grip the blade; hold the cutting edge away from you and then firmly fix it into position. Fixation by hand is not advisable and may result in injury.

2.2.2 Forceps

There are two basic types of forceps – toothed and non-toothed – which are available in different sizes. In general, toothed forceps are used to grasp skin and fascia. Non-toothed forceps are used to hold delicate tissues such as blood vessels and bowel in which there is risk of puncture.

The correct way to hold forceps is shown in Figure 2.4. The forceps are held with the non-dominant hand. Note how the tips of the forceps face the operator with the hand curved round.

2.2.3 Needle Holders

These vary in size and should be used in accordance with the depth of the wound. It is useful to ensure that the opening and closure of the holder is reasonably smooth and easy so as to avoid jerky movements. When using needle holders, check that they are not worn, otherwise the needle may slip from side to side in the jaws of the instrument, making suturing difficult.

2.2.4 Retractors

Self-retaining retractor – this is a useful instrument for holding a wound open to allow deeper dissection. Care must be taken to avoid trauma to the tissues from the "teeth" during insertion and removal of the retractor.

2 Instruments, Sutures and Diathermy 11

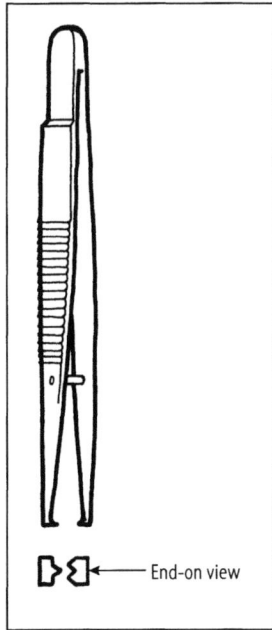

Figure 2.3. Toothed forceps

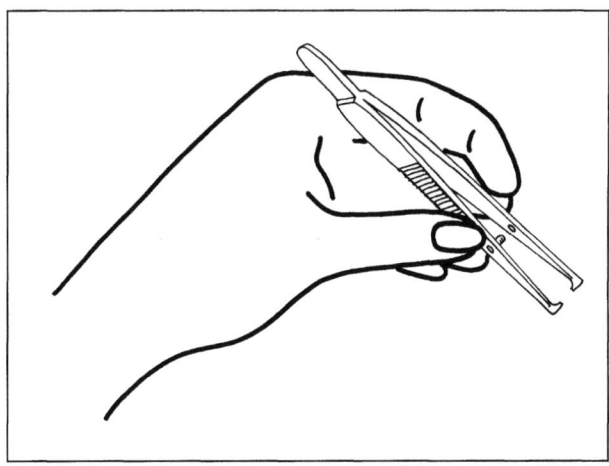

Figure 2.4. Correct way to hold forceps

Hand-held retractors of different sizes are available; these include skin hooks, "cats claws" and the Langenbeck retractor (see Figure 2.6) all of which are used to attain better exposure.

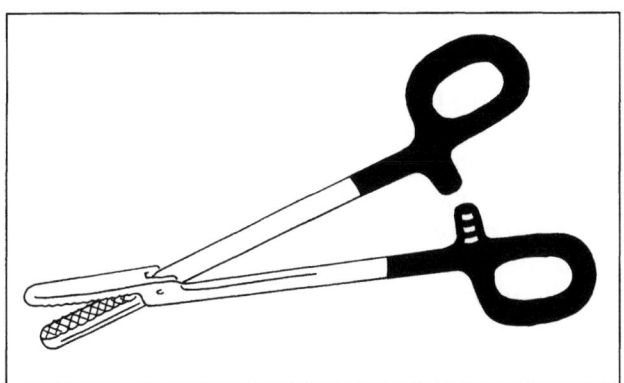

Figure 2.5. Needle holder

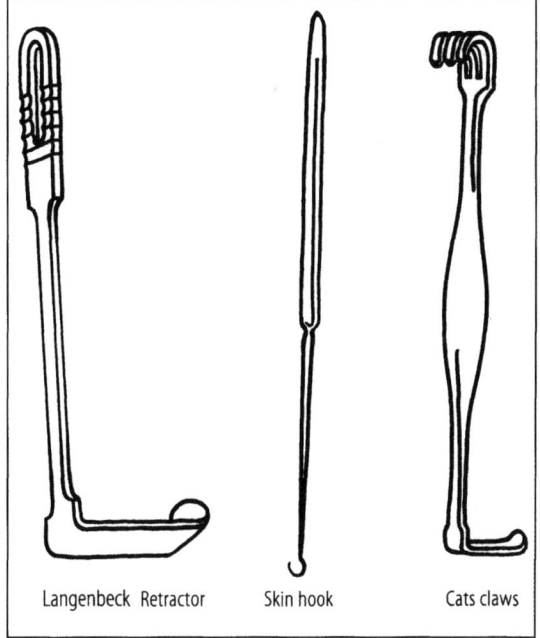

Figure 2.6. Retractors

2.2.5 Curettes

These are narrow handled instruments with spoon-shaped ends of different sizes. The edges of the "spoon" are sharp and are used to scrape the tissues. The curette can be used to clean out abscess cavities or to remove tiny naevi.

2.2.6 Infiltration Needles

In day-case surgery, four main sizes of needles are required:

- "white" $19G \times 1\frac{1}{2}''$
- "green" $21G \times 1\frac{1}{2}''$
- "blue" $23G \times 1''$
- "orange" $25G \times \frac{5}{8}''$

Use the "white" or "green" needle to draw up fluids into a syringe.

For skin infiltration the "orange" needle is least traumatic and least painful. However, only a small area can be infiltrated using it, necessitating repeated stabs if a large area is to be anaesthetised. If this is the case, then a "blue" or sometimes even a "green" needle is preferable.

Digital ring blocks are best carried out with the "blue" needle, except on the hallux where a "green" needle may be necessary.

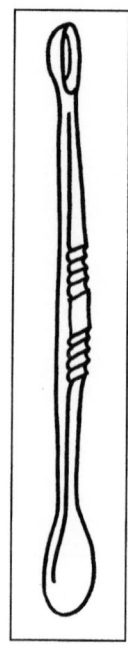

Figure 2.7.
Curette

2.2.7 Tourniquets

Tourniquets are used to restrict the blood flow to an area so that the operating field is clearly visible, for example, a wedge excision of an ingrown toe nail. A piece of rubber tubing is wrapped tightly once or twice around the base of the toe and held in arterial forceps. It should be applied after infiltration of the anaesthetic.

In some cases it is necessary to restrict blood flow to the whole limb, for example during excision of a ganglion. This is achieved by elevating the limb to drain the venous system, then applying an inflatable tourniquet to the upper portion of the limb and inflating the tourniquet to above arterial pressure (usually 200 mm Hg in the arm and 350 mm Hg in the leg). Make sure that both the inflation time and the deflation time of the tourniquet are recorded in the operation note. Also make sure that wool padding (for example Velband) is put between the skin and the tourniquet. This is to avoid nerve injury. Applying an Eschmarch band (a tough rubber "bandage" to drain the blood out of the limb before inflation of the tourniquet) is unnecessary and can lead to complications such as injury to the nerves and thus should be avoided.

2.3 Sutures

2.3.1 Principles

The choice of suture requires consideration of several properties. These include

- absorbable or non-absorbable properties
- thickness
- strength
- ease of knotting and handling
- body reaction to the material
- cost.

As well as this, a choice of needle must be made with regard to

- size
- shape
- edges
- thickness.

2.3.2 Materials

There are two main types of suture: absorbable and non-absorbable.

Absorbable sutures break down within the tissues, losing their strength over a certain period of time. They can be used to hold deep tissues together or for subcuticular suturing of the skin.

Non-absorbable sutures are permanent; they require removal if used on skin. They are also used in deeper tissues; for example, to secure a mesh in position for hernia repair. Table 2.1 below lists the most commonly used sutures today. Older types of suture material such as catgut and linen are not mentioned, as their use is declining. Sutures are graded by their diameter in tenths of a mm (except for BP sizes for catgut, which are different). Table 2.2 shows the commonly used sizes.

2.3.3 Technique

Interrupted
This is used to close the skin. The suture is subcutaneous and should be placed at equal distances from the skin edges. A reef knot is made to secure the suture.

Table 2.1. Commonly used sutures

Suture type	Period of strength (days)	Structure	Uses
Absorbable			
polyglactin (Vicryl) *	28	braided	subcutaneous, subcuticular
polydioxanone (PDS)	56	monofilament	subcutaneous, subcuticular
polyglyconate (Maxon)	30	monofilament	subcutaneous, subcuticular, fascia
Non-absorbable			
polypropylene (Prolene) *	permanent	monofilament	skin, subcuticular
polyamide (Ethilon)	permanent	monofilament	skin, subcuticular
silk	permanent	braided	skin, securing drains

* We recommend these sutures.

Table 2.2. Commonly used sizes of sutures

Size 1/10 of a mm	British Pharmacopoeia (BP) size	Use in tissues
5	2	muscle, fascia
4	1	muscle, fascia
3.5	0	fascia
3.0	2/0	subcutaneous, fascia
2.0	3/0	skin on limbs and trunk, scalp, subcutaneous
1.5	4/0	skin
1.0	5/0	face
0.7	6/0	blood vessels
0.5	7/0	eyes

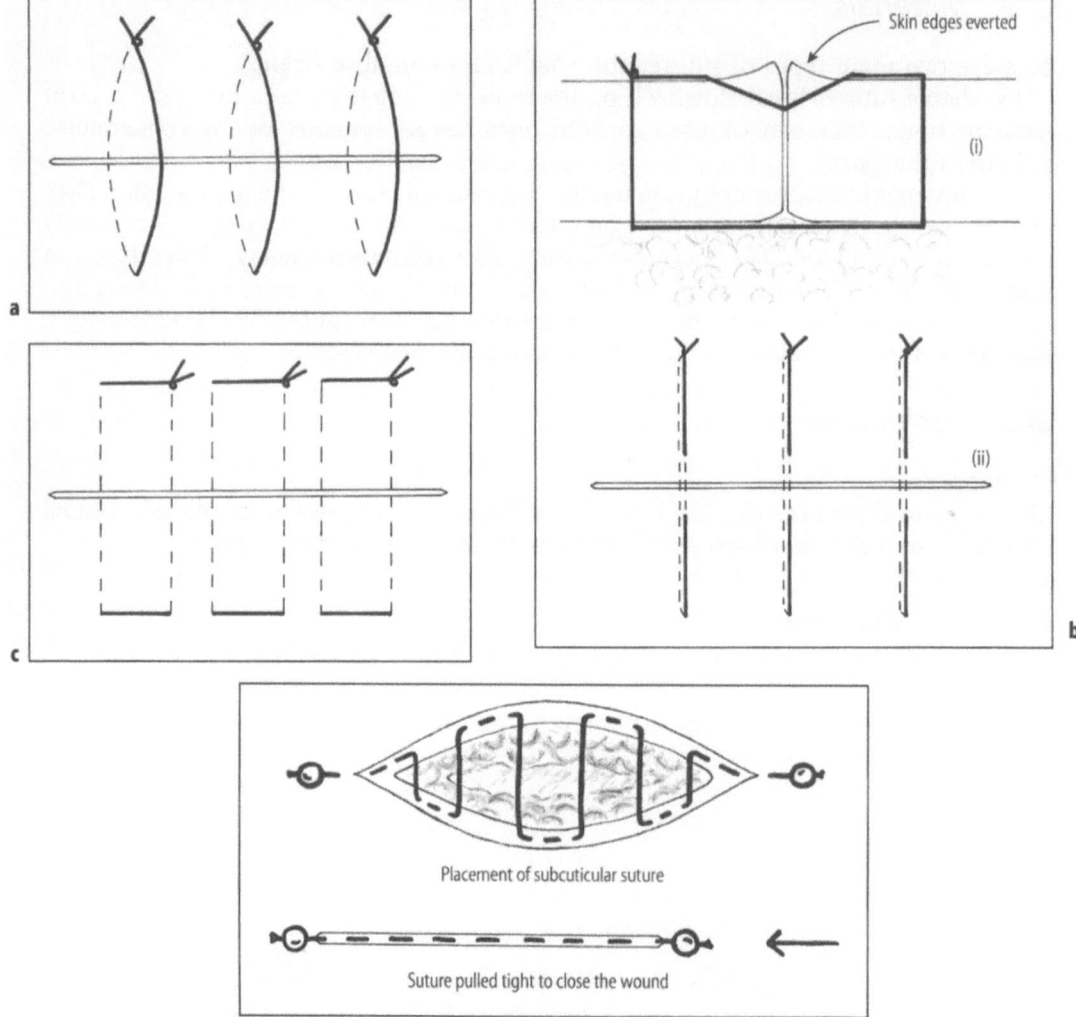

Figure 2.8. Four types of suture: **a** interrupted, **b** vertical mattress, **c** horizontal mattress and **d** subcuticular

Vertical mattress
This is used to evert the skin edges. It is useful in wounds where there may be tension in the wound. Part of the suture is within the skin (superficial) and part is deeper in the subcutaneous tissue.

Horizontal mattress
This is also used for everting edges. The suture lies in the same plane throughout.

Subcuticular
This suture produces a very neat scar that heals well, provided it is done carefully. It can only be used where there is no tension on the wound. Absorbable (for example PDS) or non-absorbable (for example Prolene) suture materials are suitable. The suture is placed along the dermal layer of the skin, starting on one side and crossing to the other and then back again, forming a ladder-like configuration. When the ends are pulled, the skin edges come together. The ends are then secured with beads or a knot.

2.3.4 Needles

Surgical needles have the suture material attached to the swage. There are many types and sizes of surgical needles. The following are the main types:

Cutting Needle
This has a triangular cross-section with sharp edges which cut through tough tissue. It is normally used to suture skin.

Round-bodied
This needle has a round cross-section and is used for suturing soft tissues which are easily penetrated, such as bowel.

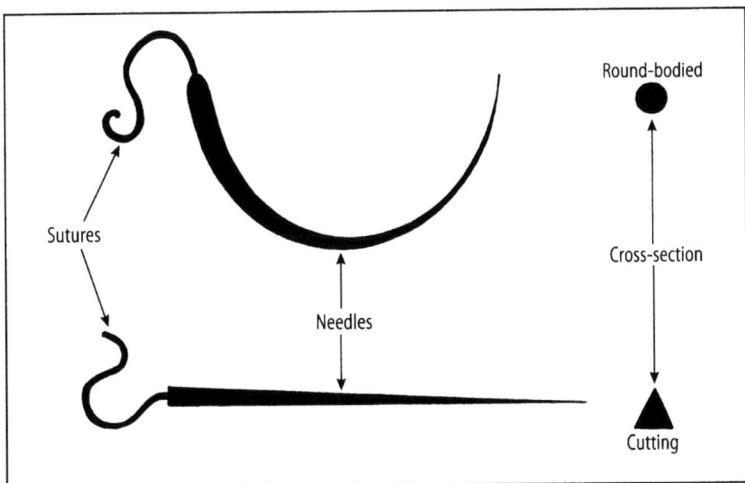

Figure 2.9. Types of needles: cutting and round-bodied

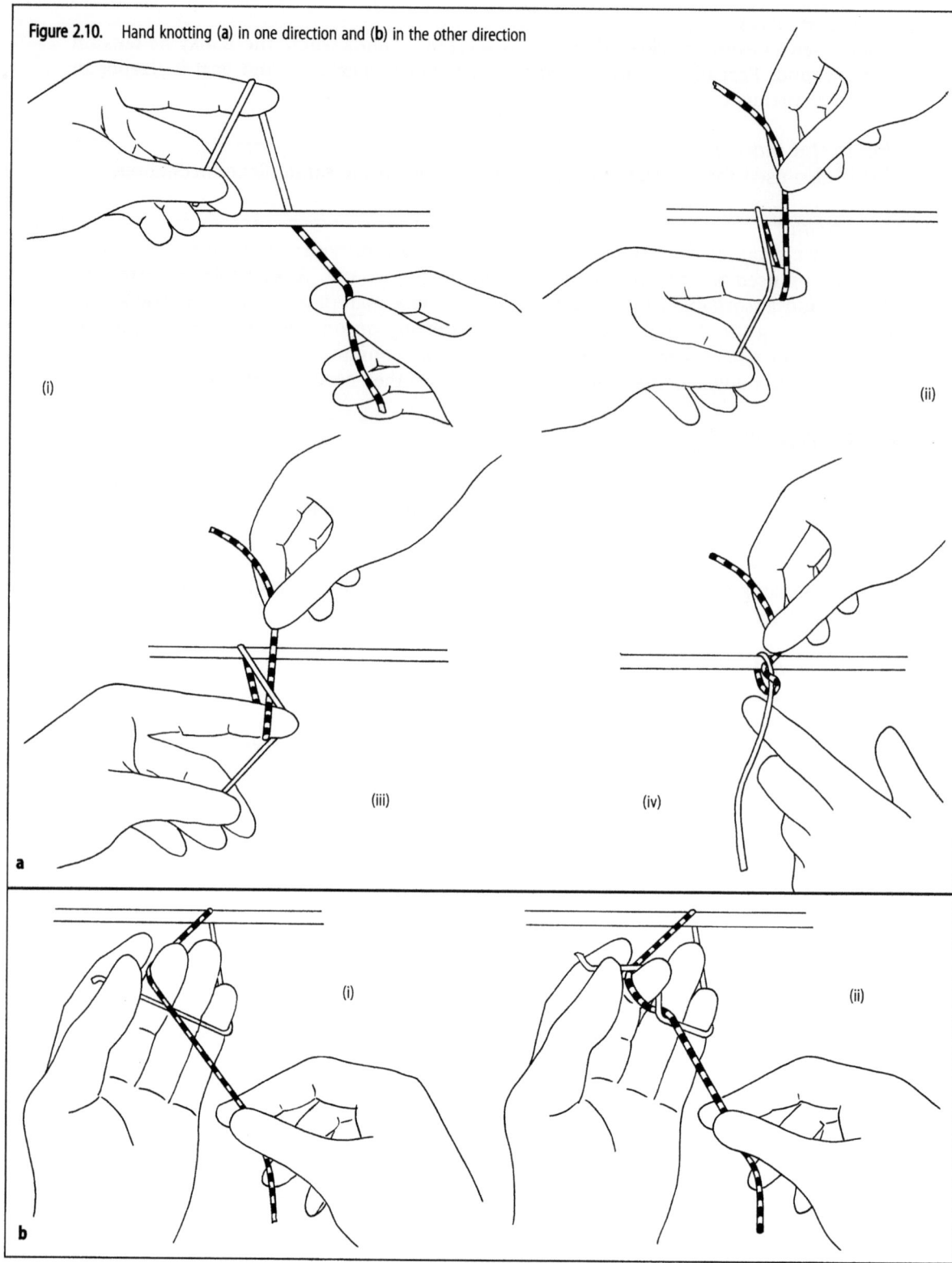

Figure 2.10. Hand knotting (a) in one direction and (b) in the other direction

Tapered Cut Needle
This has a "cutting" tip and a round cross-section, and is used for vascular surgery.

Shape
Needles used for suturing may be straight or curved. The choice depends on accessibility to the tissues and personal preference. Straight needles in general are only used for skin suturing, though curved needles may be used for this as well.

The straight needle is good for subcuticular suturing. A $^3/_8"$ circle curved needle is good for suturing skin using a simple or mattress suture technique.

2.3.5 Knots

Knots are formed using the hands or with instruments. The knot must be firm and secure so that it does not come undone. This is ensured by forming a reef knot which should lie "square". The knot should be placed on one side of the skin wound so that it does not lie in the middle of the wound and does not interfere with healing.

Hand Knotting
The standard reef knot is formed by a single throw in one direction and the next throw in the opposite direction. This is secured with further alternating throws according to the type of suture material.
For Vicryl or other braided material, use at least three throws.
For Prolene or other monofilament material, use a minimum of six throws.

Instrument Knotting
One end of the suture is wrapped around the needle holder and the other end is then pulled through the loop to form the first throw. The reef knot is completed by a second throw in the opposite direction. Further alternating throws are required to secure the knot.

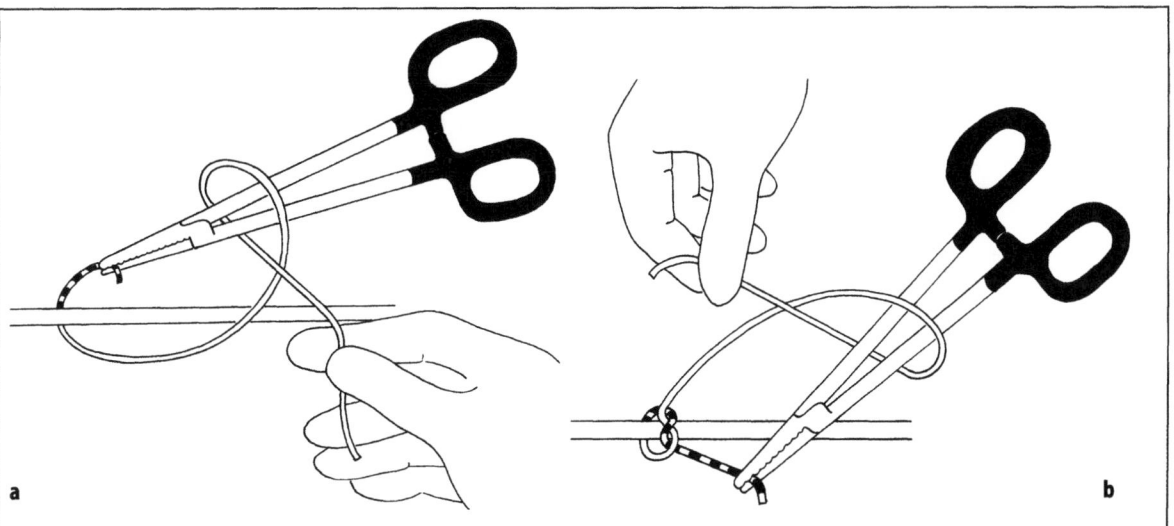

Figure 2.11. Instrument knotting

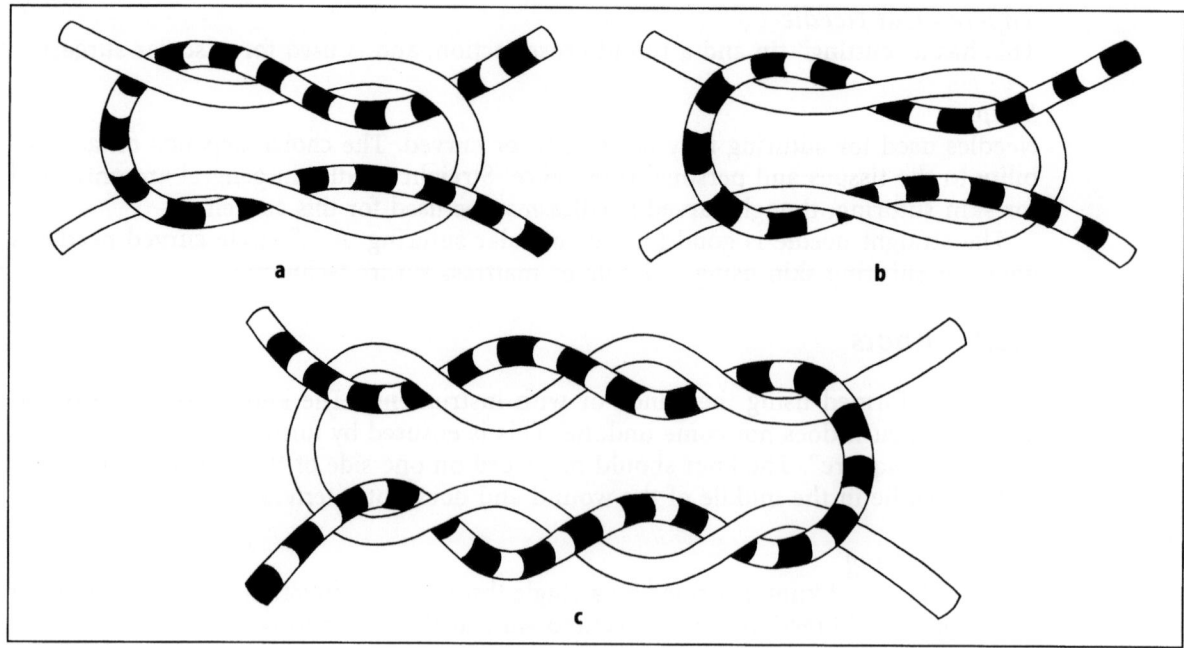

Figure 2.12. Types of knots: **a** reef, **b** sliding and **c** surgeon's knot

Sliding Knot or "Granny" Knot
When two throws are made in the same direction, the knot formed is not secure and will "slide". This can be used to tighten a knot but equally can loosen with ease and therefore must be secured with a throw in the opposite direction to form a reef knot.

Surgeon's Knot
This knot requires two hands. A double throw is placed to start with and then a double throw in the opposite direction to secure.

With an instrument, the suture is wrapped around the needle holder twice to get the double throw and secured with a double throw in the opposite direction.

2.3.6 Clips and Staples

Clips and staples are generally used for large wounds. The principles of skin closure are the same as with sutures. The edges must be approximated and everted at the same time, using a pair of toothed forceps. A disposable stapler is used to apply the clips. Removal of clips requires a special instrument and is done after the same interval as that for suture removal. The advantage in using clips or staples is in the speed of application, especially in large wounds. The main disadvantage is cost.

2.3.7 Removal of Sutures and Clips

The length of time that sutures are left in place varies in different parts of the body due to the different thickness of the skin. A general guide is:

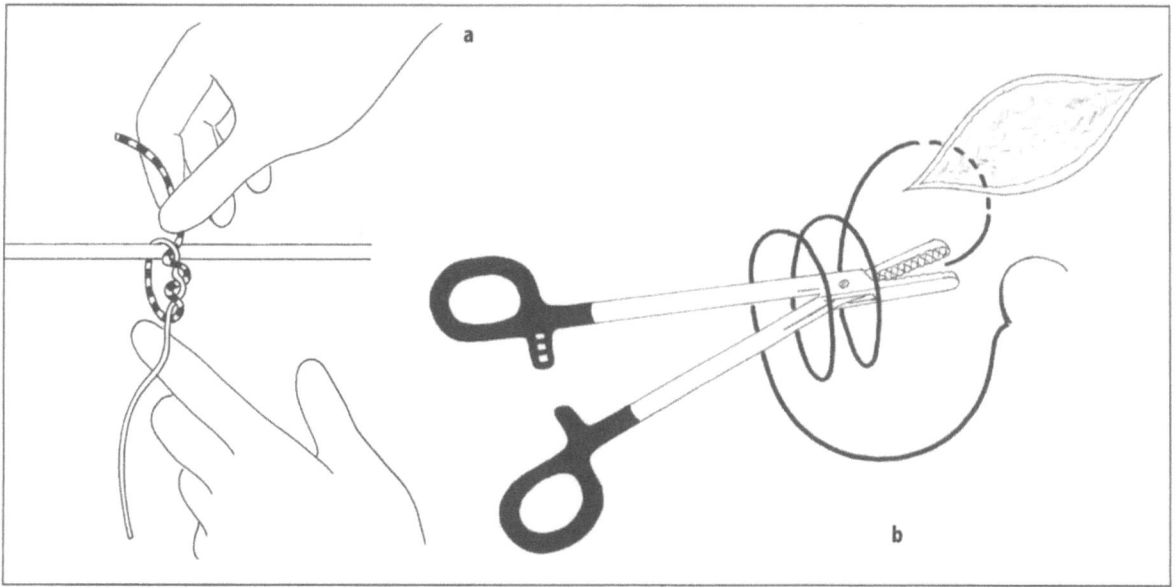

Figure 2.13. Surgeon's knot by (**a**) hand and (**b**) by instrument tying

- face – 5 days
- abdomen – 7 days
- trunk/limbs – 10 to 14 days

It is possible to remove sutures and clips earlier and then apply adhesive strips (Steristrips) to keep the wound apposed. This may be useful in areas where scarring is particularly undesirable, for example the face.

2.4 Diathermy

Diathermy is electrosurgery used to cut and coagulate tissues. It involves the passage of an electric (alternating) current via special forceps to the tissues. The concentration of current generates heat that then causes coagulation.

In minor surgery, diathermy is usually used to cauterise blood vessels to ensure haemostasis. There are two main types: monopolar and bipolar.

2.4.1 Monopolar (unipolar)

The current is produced at the tip of the forceps, which acts as the active electrode, and returns to the generator via a plate attached to the body. Therefore, good contact must be obtained between the plate and the skin, and it is important to keep the plate dry. Monopolar diathermy can be used for (1) coagulating bleeding vessels (using interrupted bursts of current) through forceps to pick up the bleeding points, or (2) cutting tissues (using a smooth sine-wave current) through a needle point instrument.

When using monopolar diathermy, it is important to ensure that no part of the patient is in contact with metal (for example part of the operating table). Otherwise, the diathermy current can "earth" or discharge through that point, possibly causing a "diathermy burn".

It is important not to use diathermy near anything flammable, for example a pool of a spirit-based antiseptic, otherwise it may combust.

Great care should also be taken if diathermy is to be used in a patient with a pacemaker, as this may interfere with its function.

Care must also be taken when using diathermy near substances able to store static electricity, as a spark may occur. The diathermy forceps or point should be kept in a container made of non-conducting material (for example a plastic quiver) when not in use during the operation, to avoid inadvertent use. Monopolar diathermy must not be used on the penis (see Section 9.7).

2.4.2 Bipolar

The current is produced down one side of the forceps, crosses the tissue to the opposite side and returns to the generator. As the current passes across the tissue, the heat causes coagulation. For good effect, the tissue is held loosely with the tips of the forceps slightly apart. Bipolar diathermy is less powerful than monopolar.

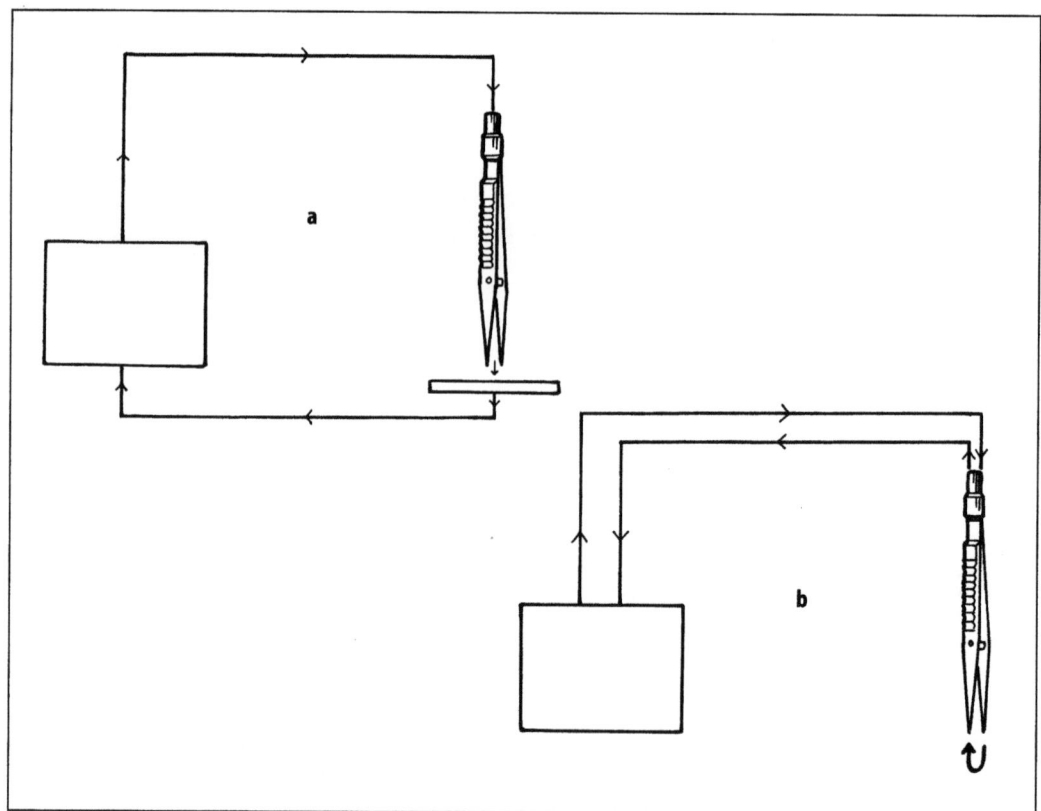

Figure 2.14. Monopolar (**a**) and bipolar (**b**) diathermy

3 Anaesthetics

3.1 Introduction

A large number of operations can be performed under local anaesthesia, especially operations on skin and subcutaneous tissue.

Sometimes, it is desirable to couple local anaesthesia with sedation such as benzodiazepines and analgesics such as Pethidine. Sedation may be given intravenously (for example Midazolam) at the time of operation or orally (for example Diazepam) about half an hour before the procedure.

If sedation, analgesia or both are given, then we recommend that the patient be monitored during the procedure (pulse, ECG, respiration, blood pressure and pulse oximetry). It may also be desirable to give the patient oxygen. It is essential to have reversal agents for the sedation (for example Flumazenil in the case of Midazolam, and Naloxone in the case of Pethidine) to hand. If neither sedation nor analgesia have been used, monitoring is not essential; however, it is prudent to have a nurse or operating department assistant (ODA) sitting next to the patient to check that the patient is well during the entire procedure.

There are a number of different types of local anaesthetics and a number of different ways of using them. These are described below.

3.2 Types of Local Anaesthetics

There are two main types of injectable local anaesthetics (LA): short-acting and long-acting. These may be plain or may be combined with Epinephrine (adrenaline) (usually 1:200,000).

3.2.1 Short-acting Local Anaesthetics

These take action quickly, but their action wears off quickly as well (usually within the hour, depending on the site). The most popular short-acting LA is Lidocaine (formally known as Lignocaine). This is available in concentrations of 0.5, 1 and 2 per cent. The higher the concentration the more the anaesthetic action. This also means that the higher the concentration, the lower the total volume that can be used safely. Therefore, if it is anticipated that a large volume of local anaesthetic is going to be needed in a procedure, the more dilute LA solution should be used. To be safe, no more than 30 ml of 1 per cent solution should be used (see Appendix B for further information). It is available either plain or combined with Epinephrine (adrenaline) (usually 1:200,000).

Epinephrine (adrenaline) prolongs the action of the LA as well as reducing bleeding from the site of operation. It does this by way of its vasoconstrictive action. It is therefore advantageous to use LA/Epinephrine (adrenaline) mixtures in highly vascular areas such as the scalp. However, it is dangerous to use Epinephrine (adrenaline) in areas supplied by end arteries, for example the digits, as distal gangrene may occur. Furthermore, if large quantities of the mixture are used or the mixture is injected intravenously by mistake, the cardiac effects of Epinephrine (adrenaline) may cause complications. If in doubt, do not use Epinephrine (adrenaline). (See Appendix B for further information on dosage.)

3.2.2 Long-acting Local Anaesthetics

These take a little longer to have effect; however, they tend to last longer (usually 2 to 3 hours). Bupivicaine (Marcaine) is such a LA. It comes in concentrations of 0.25, 0.5 and 1 per cent. It also comes either plain or combined with Epinephrine (adrenaline) (usually 1:200,000). The same precautions regarding the quantity of LA used apply to both long- and short-acting LAs. (See Appendix B for further information on dosage.)

3.2.3 Mixtures

Some surgeons use mixtures of short- and long-acting LAs to get the benefits of both, i.e. rapid onset of anaesthesia and prolonged action. We have not found this useful and recommend using a long-acting LA to prolong patient comfort following the procedure. We also recommend giving the local anaesthetic prior to formal disinfection of the area, draping and gowning, in order to give the anaesthetic more time to take action before starting the procedure.

3.2.4 Precautions

- Always ask the patient if they have had a LA in the past and whether they had any reactions to it.
- Always check the solution you are using to ensure that it is the correct one and that it is not past its expiry date. It is preferable to get another person to check this with you.
- It is important that the total amount of LA does not exceed the maximum recommended dose. Always check how much is safe to give before using LA (this will depend on patient age and weight).
- If LA with Epinephrine (adrenaline) is used, be sure not to use it in the extremities (i.e. digits, nose, ear, penis or any other areas where end arteries are the only blood supply), as distal gangrene may occur.
- If LA with Epinephrine (adrenaline) is used, make sure that the patient does not have a cardiac history and that the total quantity given is within safe margins.
- Always ensure that the LA is not given intravascularly (by withdrawing on the syringe and ensuring that no blood is drawn up before infiltration). Otherwise the cardiac affects of the LA and/or Epinephrine (adrenaline) infused may result in complications.

Another way of anaesthetising the skin without injection is by the use of ethyl chloride spray that rapidly freezes the skin, rendering it insensate. However, this is quite painful, and the anaesthetic effect is very short lived (a few minutes). Thus, this method is only useful for very short procedures such as incision and drainage of small superficial abscesses. In general, we do not feel that this is a dependable method of anaesthesia and do not recommend it.

Another way of anaesthetising the skin without injection is with the use of anaesthetic creams. These, however, do not give sufficient anaesthetic effect to perform procedures, but are usually used to anaesthetise the area of skin for an intravenous injection or for insertion of a venous cannula, especially in children.

3.3   Local Infiltration

This method of anaesthesia is useful for operations on the skin or subcutaneous tissues. Use plain 0.5 per cent Bupivicaine, unless the lesion is very big and you anticipate you will need more than 30 ml, in which case you should use 0.25 per cent plain Bupivicaine. If the area of operation is very vascular (for example the scalp) then use Bupivicaine with 1:200,000 Epinephrine (adrenaline). Epinephrine (adrenaline) also prolongs the action of the local anaesthetic. Never use Epinephrine (adrenaline) in areas supplied by end arteries, for example the digits, as distal gangrene may ensue.

- Mark the periphery of the lesion to be excised so that the dimensions of the lesion are obvious.
- Check your local anaesthetic and draw it up.
- Get rid of any air in the syringe and ensure that the solution has reached the tip of the needle by expressing a few drops.
- Use a "green" needle if a lot of LA needs to be given, a "blue" needle if a moderate amount of LA needs to be given and an "orange" needle if only a small amount of LA needs to be given.
- Warn the patient that the LA will "sting" but that this will only last for a short while.
- Clean the area to be injected with an alcohol wipe.
- Insert the needle through the skin so that the tip is just under the skin, aspirate (ensure that no blood is aspirated) and inject the LA. This should raise a visible "bleb" in the skin.
- Advance the needle, aspirate and inject more.
- Keep on doing this until the whole of the area of the lesion as well as a reasonable distance beyond it has been infiltrated. You may need to re-insert the needle in a different position in order to cover a wide area.
- If the lesion is subcutaneous then you will also need to infiltrate the same area at a deeper level.
- Wait a few minutes until the LA has taken effect.
- Check that the area has been effectively anaesthetised by pricking the area with a needle before you proceed with the operation.
- Keep more LA at hand in case you need more during the procedure.

24 Manual of Ambulatory General Surgery

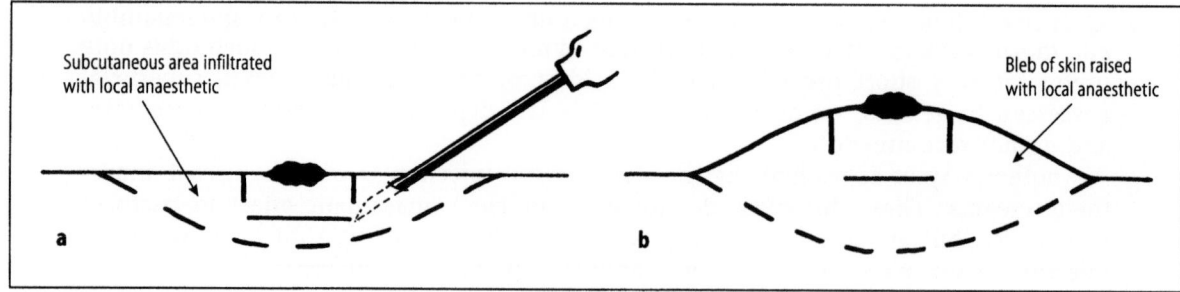

Figure 3.1. LA infiltration

3.4 Ring Block

This method of anaesthesia is useful for procedures on the fingers or toes. Use plain 0.5 per cent Bupivicaine, **never** with Epinephrine (adrenaline). The principle of this technique relies on the fact that the digital nerves are the only sensory supply to the fingers and toes and they run in very close proximity to the proximal phalanx on either side of each digit. Injecting LA in this area results in anaesthesia to the whole digit.

- Prepare the local anaesthetic and clean the skin as described earlier.
- Insert the needle into the skin at the base in the middle of the finger or toe so that the tip is just under the skin, aspirate (ensure that no blood is aspirated) and inject the LA. This should raise a visible "bleb" in the skin.

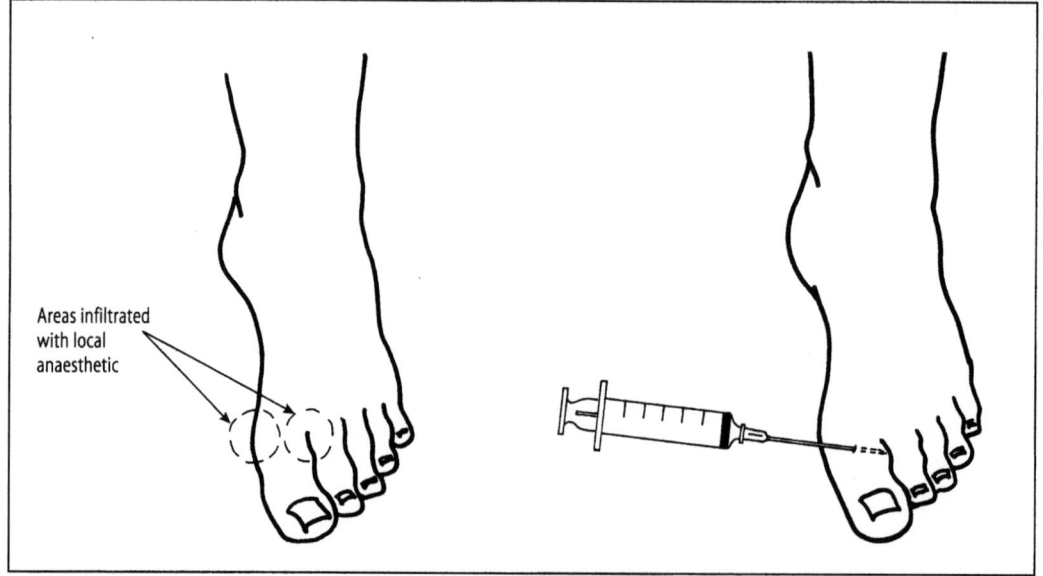

Figure 3.2. Ring block

- Advance the needle deep and laterally. You should try and aim the needle so that it is in very close proximity to the proximal phalanx. Keep advancing the needle until you are almost out on the other side.
- Now very slowly pull the needle back out while injecting the LA at the same time.
- Keep doing this until the needle is almost out.
- You should see swelling of the side of the digit and the web space.
- Repeat the same procedure for the other side of the digit (medially).
- In the hallux, you will also need to inject subcutaneously transversely on the dorsal and volar aspects of the toe.
- Now place a tourniquet around the toe (for example a thin rubber catheter) and secure it using a mosquito or Dunhill artery clip.
- Wait a few minutes until the LA has taken action.
- Check that the area has been effectively anaesthetised by pricking the area with a needle before you proceed with the operation.
- Keep more LA at hand in case you need more during the procedure.

3.5 Nerve Block

This method of anaesthesia is useful for procedures on areas supplied by a small number of sensory nerves (usually a maximum of three) for example the foot. Only use plain 0.5 per cent Bupivicaine. The principle of this technique is that the sensory nerves are infiltrated with LA in predictable anatomic locations. This results in anaesthesia to the whole area supplied by the nerve. These are advanced techniques and are beyond the scope of this manual. More information can be found in texts on regional anaesthesia.

4 Vascular Access

4.1 Introduction

Haemorrhage with hypovolaemia is a common cause of "shock". The treatment of this is volume replacement via two large-bore cannulae sited in peripheral veins. As peripheral blood vessels constrict to maintain the central circulation, the veins collapse and it may be impossible to gain venous access by direct venepuncture. It will then be necessary to perform a venous cutdown.

A central line should not be used for volume replacement as the cannula is long and narrow, and therefore the flow is not rapid. However, it is used in the emergency situation when peripheral access is not achieved. A central line is far more useful to monitor central venous pressure (CVP) and also for total parenteral nutrition (TPN). In children, an interosseous needle can be used for fluid replacement.

4.2 Venous Cutdown

Venous cutdown is performed on the long saphenous vein at the ankle, just anterior and superior to the medial malleolus. It is sometimes possible to see a venous gutter at this point.

Objective To gain venous access.
Indication Hypovolaemic "shock" with no access to peripheral blood veins.
Setting Aseptic conditions and technique.
Preparation Cleanse the skin over the medial aspect of the ankle with antiseptic solution, e.g. chlorhexidine.
Drape the ankle exposing the medial malleolus and surrounding area.
Anaesthetic Local – plain Lidocaine 1 per cent.
Infiltrate the skin over the vein with about 2 ml of local anaesthetic.

Procedure

- Make a transverse incision through the skin overlying the vein.
- If the vein cannot be seen, make a transverse incision of 2 cm length just above and in front of the medial malleolus.
- If possible, use a small self-retaining retractor or, if you have an assistant, use "cats' claws" retractors or "skin hooks" to keep the wound open.

28 Manual of Ambulatory General Surgery

- Dissect down carefully until the long saphenous vein is seen. If difficulty in finding the vein is encountered, extend the incision.
- Use arterial forceps to dissect and free the vein from adjacent tissue.
- Expose about 2 cm of the vein.
- Using a Vicryl tie (3/0), fold it in half and pass it under the vein. Divide the suture at the halfway mark so that there are now two lengths around the vein. Tie the distal (caudal) suture securely. Leave the ends long to allow you to pull up on the vein.
- Make a small transverse incision on the vein to gain access.
- Introduce a plastic cannula into the vein and secure this by tying the proximal (cephaloid) suture around the vein and cannula.
- Cut the ends of the silk ties leaving a "tail" of about 5 mm.
- Attach the intravenous giving-set to administer fluids.
- Close the incision with interrupted 3/0 Prolene sutures.
- Apply a transparent adhesive dressing.

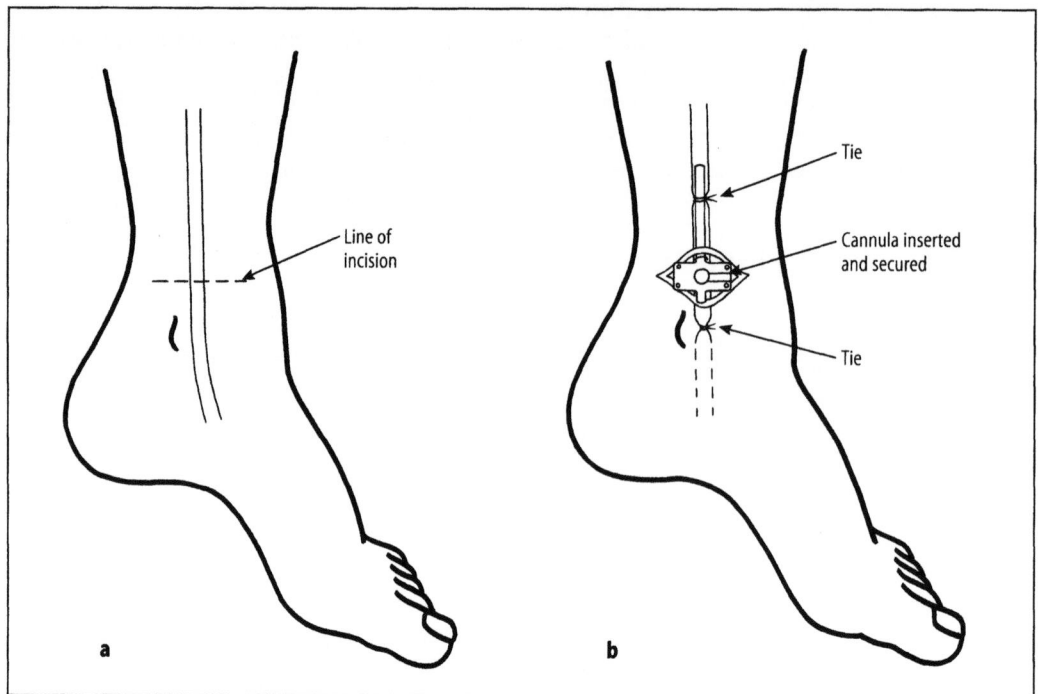

Figure 4.1. Venous cutdown: incision (**a**), and cannula *in situ* (**b**)

4.3 Central Lines

Central venous access means access to the superior vena cava or right atrium. It can be gained via the subclavian or internal jugular veins (occasionally it may be necessary to gain access through the femoral vein). The technique used is the "Seldinger" technique

– it is important that this technique is fully understood to avoid any mishaps. Essentially, a large-bore needle attached to a syringe is used to puncture the vein, at the same time aspirating on the syringe. Aspiration of blood confirms entry into the vein. The syringe is then detached from the needle. A guidewire is fed into the needle for an estimated distance and the needle removed. The cannula is then inserted over the guidewire. Care should be taken to hold on to the guidewire so that it does not slip into the circulation! Once the cannula is in place, the guidewire is removed and the cannula is secured in position.

There are two types of cannulae: single lumen or triple lumen. The choice depends on the number of access ports required.

Objective To gain central venous access.
Indications To monitor CVP and fluid management.
 To administer TPN.
 To administer drugs directly to the heart or superior vena cava.
 Occasionally, to administer fluids.
Setting Aseptic technique.
 There is a significant risk of infection, so the entire procedure should be done with great care using sterile equipment.

4.3.1 Subclavian Vein Access

Position Supine with about 20 degrees of head-down tilt to distend the veins and prevent air embolism. Turn the head away from the side of entry.
Preparation Clean a wide area of skin with iodine, over the clavicle on the side of entry. Drape the area to create a sterile field.
Anaesthetic Local – Lidocaine 1 per cent.
 Infiltrate the skin just below the clavicle at the point where it curves, i.e. at the junction between the outer and middle two-thirds.

Procedure

- Introduce the needle 0.5 cm below the clavicle, at the junction between the outer and middle two-thirds of the clavicle, and pointing towards the suprasternal notch.
- Advance the needle posteriorly behind the clavicle to enter the subclavian vein. Withdraw on the syringe at the same time so that a flow of blood into the syringe indicates entry into the vein.
- Ensure that this is venous and not arterial blood. Venous blood is darker. If in doubt disconnect the syringe from the needle momentarily and observe the flow of blood from the hub of the needle. If it is bright red and pulsating then it is likely that you are in the subclavian artery and not vein. In this case remove the needle and start again.
- Advance the needle a further 1 or 2 mm. Check that you can still aspirate blood. Remove the syringe leaving the needle in place and cover the end to prevent air embolism and blood loss.
- Insert the guidewire through the needle for a length of about 15 cm and then remove the needle.

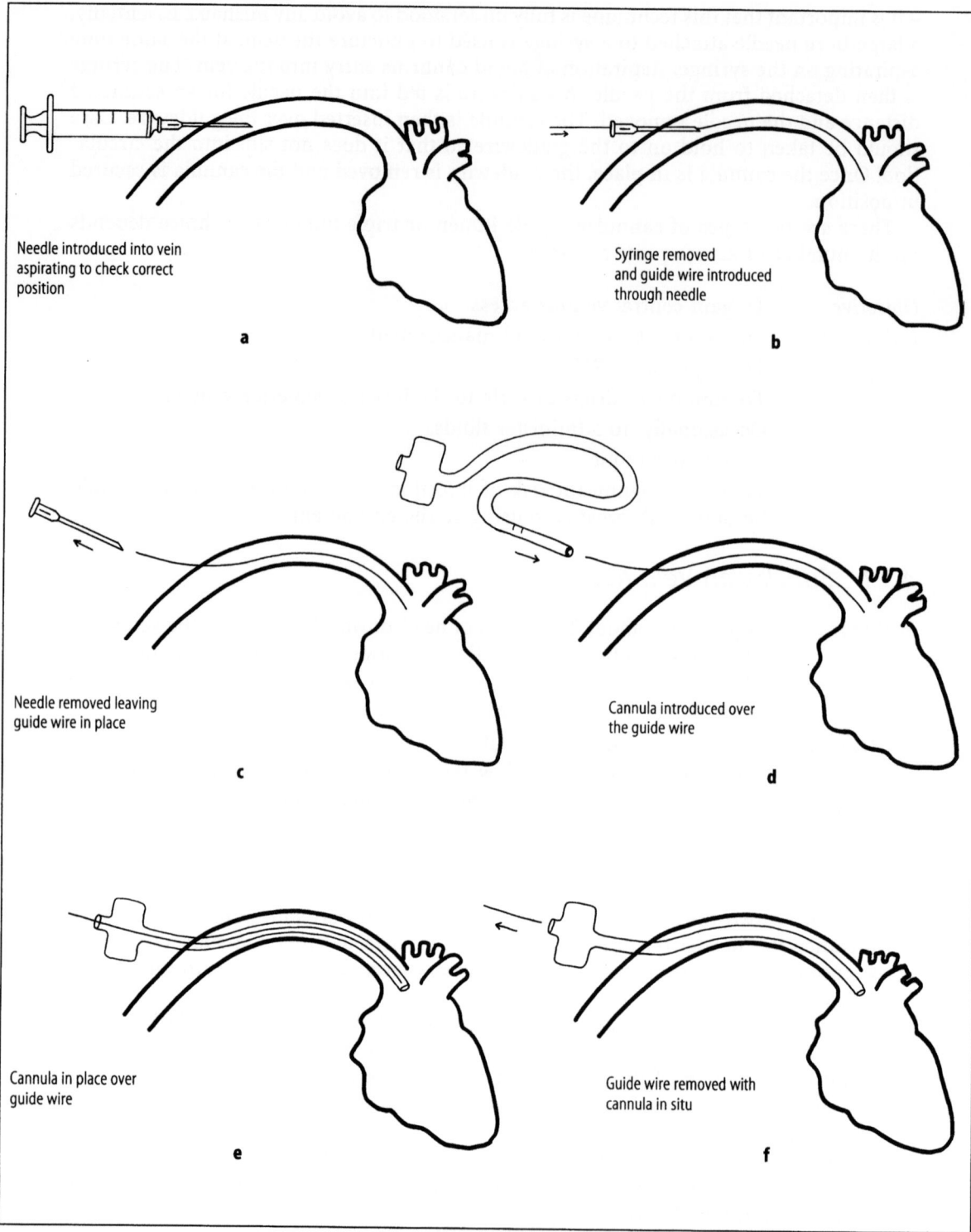

Figure 4.2. "Seldinger" technique for insertion of central lines

- If there is any resistance to the passage of the guidewire or cannula (see Figure 4.3) try abducting the arm of the patient on that side. This tends to straighten the vein. If you still have difficulty, then it will be necessary to remove the guidewire, connect the syringe to the needle and ensure that you are still in the vein (by aspirating blood). If you are not sure you are in the vein, then you need to start again.
- It may be necessary to use a plastic dilator over the guidewire or to make a small incision in the skin to allow the entry of the cannula.
- Slide the cannula over the guidewire. The guidewire outside the skin should be kept long enough to allow you to slide the cannula over it completely before the cannula starts entering through the skin incision.
- Hold the free end of the guidewire beyond the cannula while you insert the cannula into the vein. This is to stop the guidewire being pushed into the vein and disappearing into the circulation!!
- Secure the cannula in place with a silk suture.
- Cover with adhesive transparent dressing.
- Obtain a chest X-ray to check the position of the cannula before use (it should be in the superior vena cava, and not curled up in the right atrium).

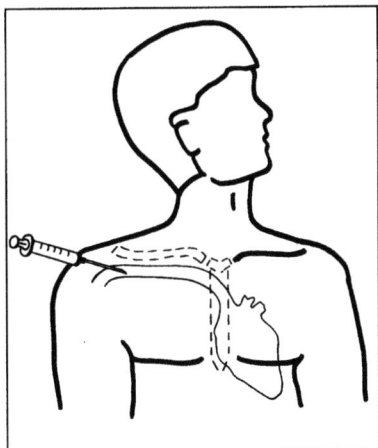

Figure 4.3.
Subclavian line

4.3.2 Internal Jugular Vein Access

Position Supine with about 20 degrees of head-down tilt to distend the veins and prevent air embolism. Turn the head away from the side of entry.

Preparation Clean the right side of the neck with iodine and then drape the area to create a sterile field.

Anaesthetic Local – Lidocaine 1 per cent
Infiltrate the skin between the two heads of sternocleidomastoid muscle.

Procedure
- Palpate the carotid artery – the vein is situated lateral to it.
- Introduce the needle through the skin at an angle of about 45 degrees, at the apex of the two heads of sternocleidomastoid muscle.

- Point the needle slightly laterally and posteriorly towards the ipsilateral nipple. Withdraw on the syringe at the same time so that a flow of blood indicates entry into the vein.
- Ensure that this is venous and not arterial blood. Venous blood is darker. If in doubt disconnect the syringe from the needle momentarily and observe the flow of blood from the hub of the needle. If it is bright red and pulsating then it is likely that you are in an artery and not the vein. In this case, remove the needle apply pressure to the area for a minimum of 5 minutes and start again.
- Once inside the vein, advance the needle a further 1 to 2 mm. Check that you are still in the vein by aspirating blood. Remove the syringe, leaving the needle in place, and cover the end to prevent air embolism and blood loss.
- Insert the guidewire through the needle an estimated distance to the superior vena cava and then remove the needle.
- The rest of the procedure is as for the subclavian vein access described in Section 4.3.1. However, you do not need to advance the catheter as much as for a subclavian line, as the distance from your entry point to the superior vena cava in the jugular approach is shorter.

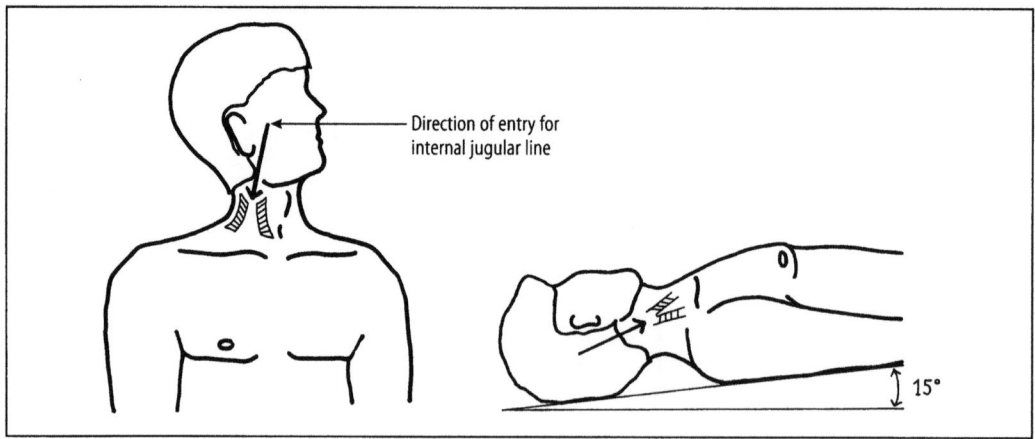

Figure 4.4. Internal jugular line

4.4 Total Parenteral Nutrition and Tunnelled Venous Lines

Total parenteral nutrition (TPN) preparations are irritant to veins and cause phlebitis. If required for only 24 to 48 hours, direct access into a peripheral vein can be used, for example in the antecubital fossa, with a large-bore cannula. It is possible to provide TPN for longer periods of time by resiting the cannula every 48 hours. However, this is not very practical and is disliked by patients. Long peripheral lines that can be inserted into an antecubital fossa with the tip of the line lying in a central vein are available. However, because of the small bore of the tubing and the length of the line, it is not possible to infuse large amounts of fluid and is therefore unpractical for long-term TPN. Central "tunnelled" lines are used for long-term TPN. A "tunnelled" line for TPN or other uses (delivery of cytotoxics, for example) should be performed by a specialist in order to avoid complications, and is not a suitable procedure for a "beginner".

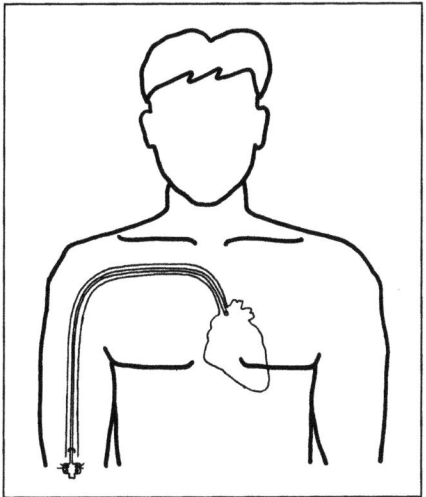

Figure 4.5. Peripheral feeding venous line *in situ*

other uses (delivery of cytotoxics, for example) should be performed by a specialist in order to avoid complications, and is not a suitable procedure for a "beginner".

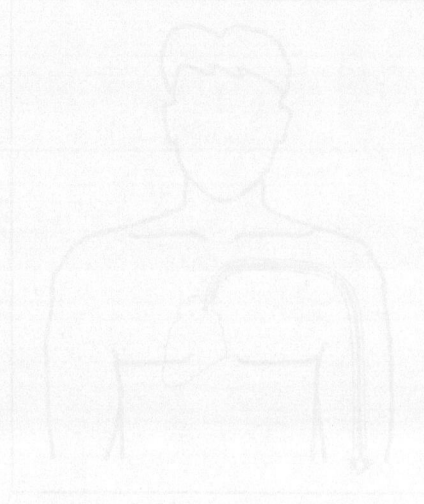

Figure 15. Patient of flexion work, the in tip.

5 Lesions of the Skin and Subcutaneous Tissue

5.1 Introduction

Most skin lesions are fairly small and can be removed under local anaesthetic. They are, therefore, ideal for day-case surgery. The skin requires suitable preparation with antiseptic solution, after which the lesion is excised (ideally in one piece), and then the wound is closed to achieve a neat cosmetically acceptable scar.

5.2 Lacerations

Lacerations occur in all sorts of settings on any part of the body.

5.2.1 Suturing Lacerations

Objective   To appose the skin edges to enhance healing (preferably by primary intention).

Indication   Injury where skin continuity is breached and a gap exists between skin edges. If the wound is small then the edges can be approximated using tissue glue or adhesive strips (Steristrips) – see Section 5.2.2.2 for details. However, in larger wounds, the wound will need to be closed using sutures.

Setting   Operating theatre/sterile conditions.

Preparation   Iodine or chlorhexidine.
Access to diathermy if the wound is bleeding.

Anaesthetic   Local.

Position   The patient should be positioned to maximise exposure of the area whilst maintaining comfort. This is important as the procedure is carried out under local anaesthetic, and the patient will need to maintain position for the duration of the procedure. It is useful to use arm boards/supports whenever necessary. A good light source is also invaluable.

Procedure

- It may be necessary to trim the edges of the skin to form a neat scar which can then heal by primary intention. Debridement of dirty wounds is very important. Do this by cutting away all non-viable tissue and cleaning the wound with copious amounts

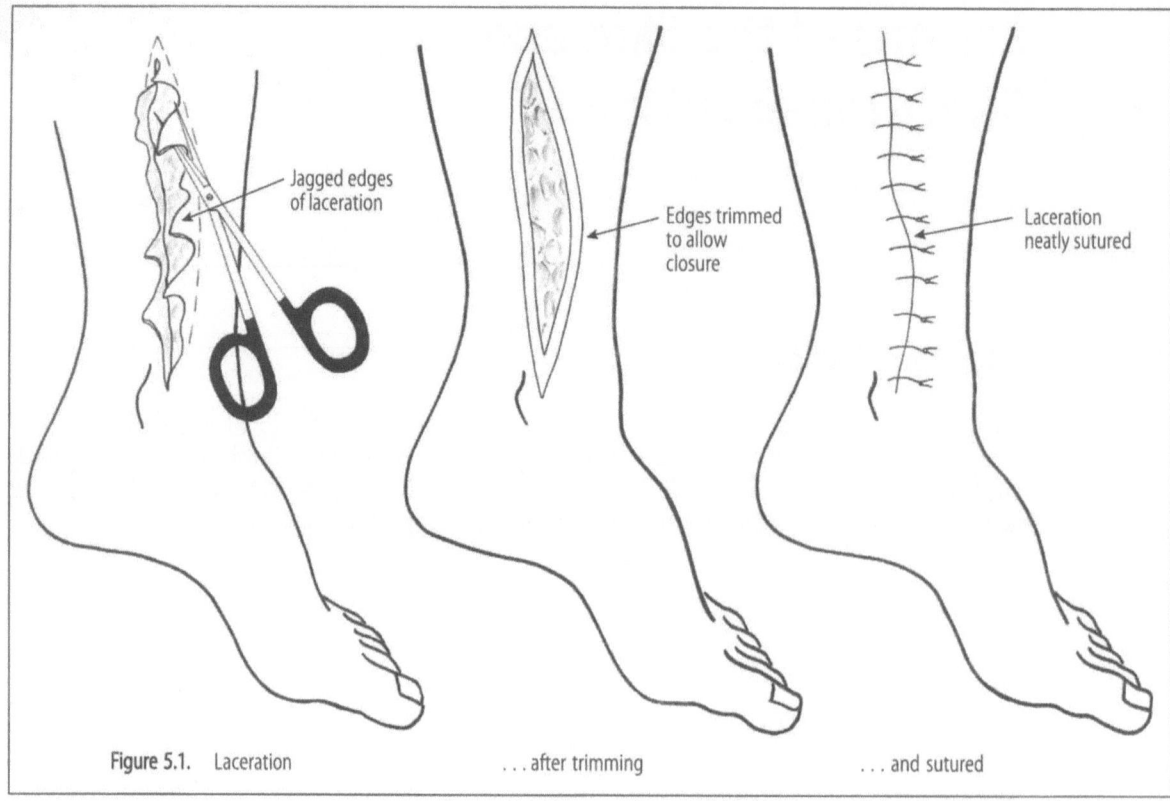

Figure 5.1. Laceration ...after trimming ...and sutured

of normal saline. An antiseptic solution such as chlorhexidine can be used. Hydrogen peroxide is also useful if there is the possibility of contamination by anaerobic organisms. (Note that in the case of compound fractures, wounds which are more than 4 hours old, and very dirty wounds, closure of the wound is not recommended.)

- Use simple sutures or mattress sutures to close the wound. Interrupted sutures should be used in dirty wounds to allow drainage of pus by removal of some of the sutures, should an infection occur.
- Op-site dressing/dry dressing is suitable for cover, to protect the wound and prevent further contamination. (Note: ensure the patient has received tetanus vaccination, and that for compound fractures and dirty wounds, a course of broad-spectrum antibiotics should be given.)
- Sutures should be removed when the healing process is well under way. A general guide for time of removal of sutures is
  - face, scalp – 5 days
  - abdomen – 7 days
  - trunk and limbs – 10 to 14 days.

5.2.2 Other Methods of Closing Skin Lacerations

5.2.2.1 "Glue"
Small lacerations, especially in children, are amenable to closure with a cyanoacrylate glue. This avoids the use of anaesthetic. The principle is to appose the skin edges accu-

rately and then place 1 or 2 drops of "glue" at one end of the wound. The glue tends to spread itself along the crevice. The skin edges should be held together for 30 seconds to 1 minute, by which time they are bonded. Care should be taken not to get any glue on the hands of the operator, otherwise you will get stuck to the patient!!

5.2.2.2 Adhesive Strips

Minor lacerations can be repaired with adhesive strips (such as Steristrips) simply to appose skin edges and hold them together. The wound must be cleaned. The surrounding skin should also be cleaned and then dried thoroughly to allow the strips to stick adequately. This may be helped by the use of tincture of benzoin applied to intact skin, as it enhances adhesion. This method is not suitable if there is tension in the wound.

5.2.3 Special Cases

5.2.3.1 Pretibial Lacerations

These occur over the shin, especially in elderly patients in whom the skin is very thin and fragile. Usually a flap of skin is raised which needs to be stretched over the wound. The flap can be secured with sutures if there is minimal tension. Otherwise adhesive strips are suitable. A small gap between the flap and the opposite edge of the wound is acceptable.

5.3 Skin Tag and Papilloma

These lesions are attached to the skin by a pedicle and need to be excised at the base.

Objective	To remove the lesion.
Indications	Cosmetic or due to repeated trauma, or "awkward" position.
Setting	Operating theatre/sterile conditions.
Position	Obtain good exposure.
Preparation	Cleanse the skin with iodine.
Anaesthetic	Local.
	Infiltrate the skin at the base of the lesion.

Procedure

- Small lesions: lift the lesion, pulling it away from the skin. Use a scalpel to cut straight across the narrow base, incorporating a small amount of normal skin.
- Large lesions: make an elliptical incision around the base of the lesion. Excise the lesion by lifting the edge of the skin with toothed forceps and cutting the skin away from subcutaneous fat with a scalpel.
- Send the removed specimen for histology. (If several lesions are removed at the same time, each specimen must be sent in a different pot with a clear indication of where it was removed from. This is to ensure that if one of the specimens needs further treatment, for example in the case of incomplete excision of a malignant lesion, then the original location of the lesion is known.

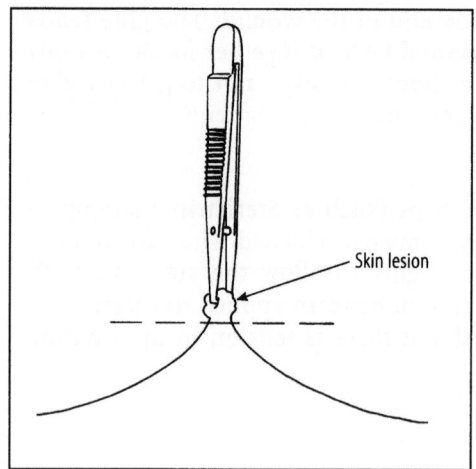 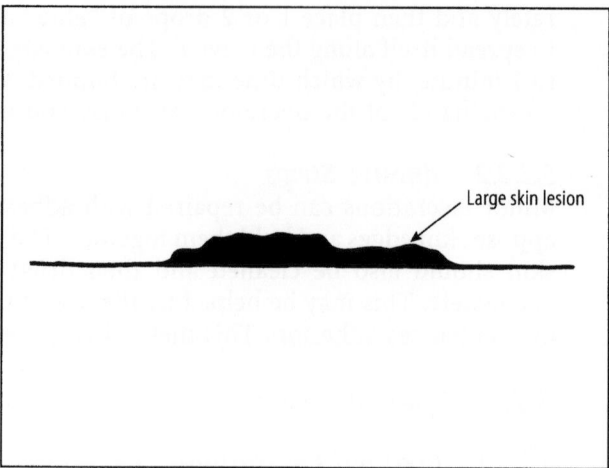

Figure 5.2. Small and large lesions

- Close the wound using 3/0 Prolene interrupted sutures.
- Cover with a dry dressing.

Post-op Remove the sutures after 5 to 7 days.

5.4 Sebaceous Cyst

A sebaceous cyst is a cutaneous structure, usually spherical in shape, which is not fixed to the underlying tissue but is fixed to skin. It usually has a punctum, although this may not be central.

Objective To excise the cyst in its entirety.

Indications Recurrent infection/inflammation.
Awkward position of the cyst resulting in trauma or irritation, for example on the scalp when combing the hair.

Setting Operating theatre/sterile conditions.

Position Position the patient to maximise exposure of the area. Ensure that the patient is comfortable.

Anaesthetic
- Local – use local anaesthetic with Epinephrine (adrenaline) if on the scalp.
- It is worthwhile marking out the position and extent of the cyst with an indelible marker prior to infiltration.
- Firstly, infiltrate the deep tissue surrounding the cyst.
- Then infiltrate the skin just over the cyst. Whilst the anaesthetic is taking effect, take the opportunity to don a gown and gloves.

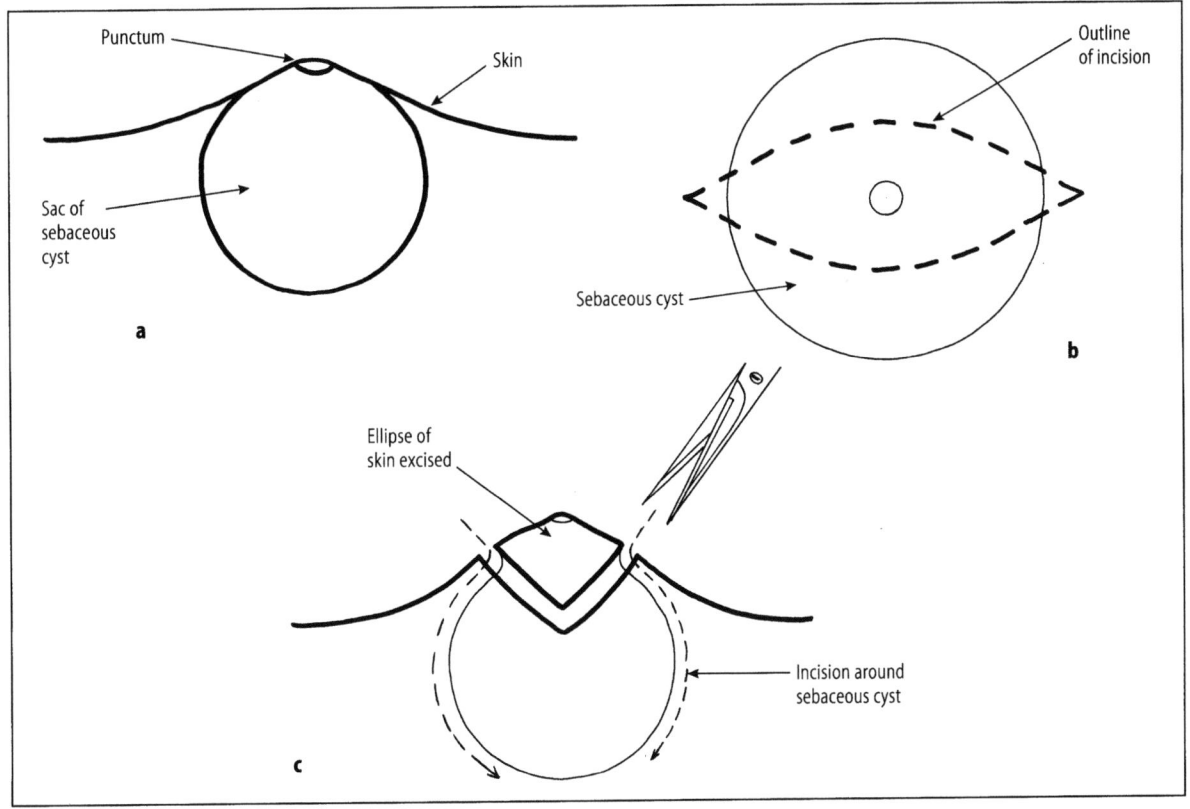

Figure 5.3. Removal of sebaceous cyst

Procedure

- Disinfect and drape the area.
- Make an elliptical incision over the cyst, encompassing the punctum.
- The length of the ellipse should be about 1.5 times the diameter of the lesion; the width of the ellipse should be just less than the diameter of the lesion.
- The incision does not need to extend around the cyst but should allow access around it.
- Using scissors or scalpel dissect out the cyst, creating a plane between it and surrounding tissue.
- Remove the cyst and attached overlying ellipse of skin. If the cyst is ruptured, it is necessary to excise the capsule, otherwise recurrence may ensue.
- Send for histology.
- Close the wound with everting sutures, i.e. interrupted simple or mattress sutures.
- Suture removal should be requested as appropriate for the site (see Section 2.3).

5.5 Dermoid Cyst

These can be removed in the same way as sebaceous cysts (see Section 5.4). If small, the cyst can be removed through a small incision by extrusion.

5.6 Lipoma

A lipoma is subcutaneous. The overlying skin is mobile and the lipoma is not fixed to underlying tissue.

Objective   To excise the lipoma.
Indications   Cosmetic.
                 Awkward site, resulting in repeated trauma or pain.
Setting   Operating theatre/sterile conditions.
Position   Position the patient to maximise exposure of the area. Ensure that the patient is comfortable.
Anaesthetic
- Local.
- It is worthwhile marking out the position and extent of the lipoma with an indelible marker prior to infiltration.
- First, infiltrate the deep tissue surrounding the lipoma. Then infiltrate the skin just over it. While the anaesthetic is taking effect, take the opportunity to don a gown and gloves.

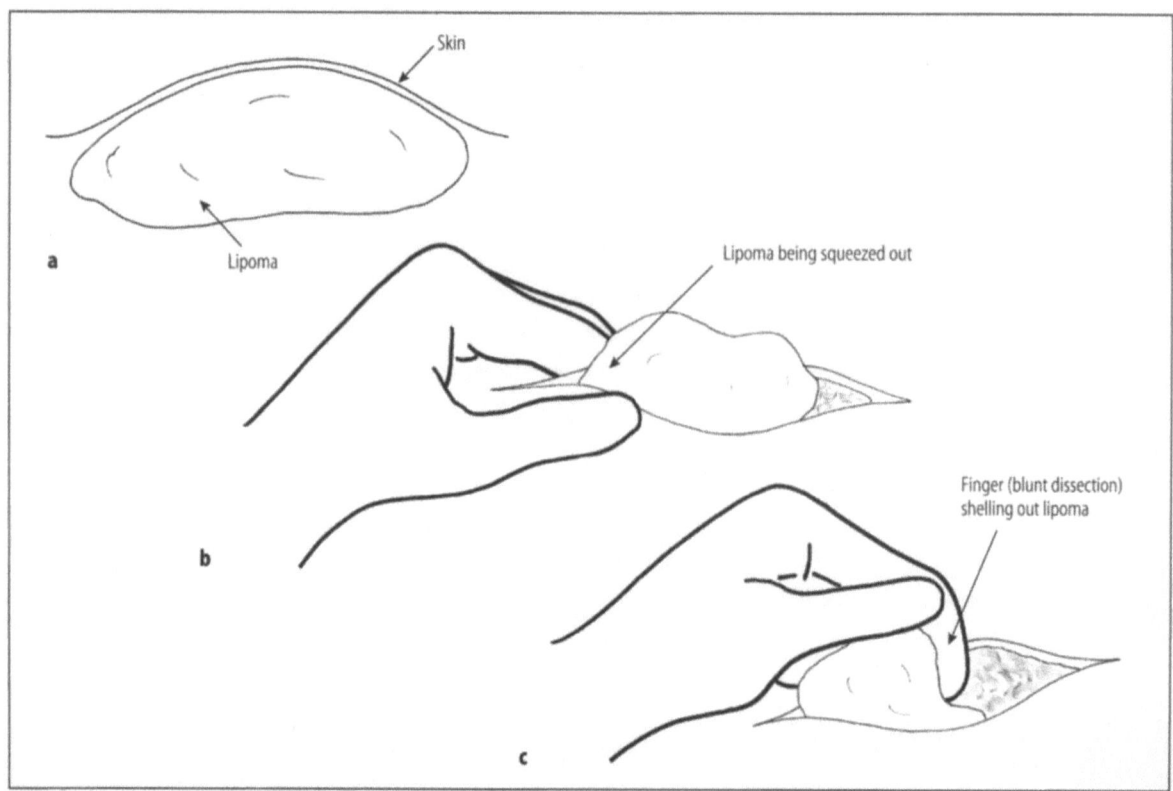

Figure 5.4. Lipoma (**a**) being squeezed out (**b**) . . . and being enucleated (**c**)

Procedure
- Cleanse the skin with an antiseptic solution.
- Make an incision along a skin crease or along Langer's lines. Start off with an incision that is about one-third the diameter of the lesion.
- The scalpel should penetrate the skin and subcutaneous fat over the lipoma. The lipoma can easily be distinguished as the colour and texture differs from that of subcutaneous fat.
- Often, it is possible to squeeze out the lipoma through such an incision. Pinch the skin on either side of the lipoma with your fingers and attempt to squeeze the lipoma out. See Figure 5.4.
- If this does not work and the incision is long enough, use a finger to enucleate (shell out) the lipoma (extend the incision further if needed). See Figure 5.4.
- If this also does not work, using scissors, divide adjacent fibrous tissue as necessary (extend the incision further if needed).
- Remove the lipoma and send for histology.
- In some instances, lipomas can be very large. In such cases, where a large area is dissected, bleeding tends to ensue and fill the cavity. It would be wise to leave in a corrugated drain or small suction drain, which can be removed 24 hours later. A compression dressing may be required to avoid haematoma formation.
- Close the wound (interrupted, mattress or subcuticular sutures).
- Remove sutures as appropriate (see Section 2.3).

5.7 Pigmented Naevus

Objective	To remove the entire lesion.
Indications	A change in the lesion, e.g. bleeding, itching, etc. (suggesting a risk of malignant change).
	Localised inflammation/trauma.
Setting	Operating theatre/sterile conditions.
Preparation	Mark out the lesion if not easily seen.
	Prepare skin with antiseptic solution.
	Have access to diathermy.
Anaesthetic	Local
Position	Position the patient to maximise exposure of the area. Ensure that the patient is comfortable.

Procedure
- Make an elliptical incision encompassing the entire lesion with at least a 1 to 2 mm margin beyond the lesion down to subcutaneous tissue (until you see the subcutaneous fat). See Figure 5.5.
- The length of the incision should be about three times the length of the lesion so that the skin edges can be easily apposed after removal.
- If possible, use a skin crease or Langer's lines.
- Pick up the skin inside the ellipse at one end with toothed forceps and free the corner. See Figure 5.5.

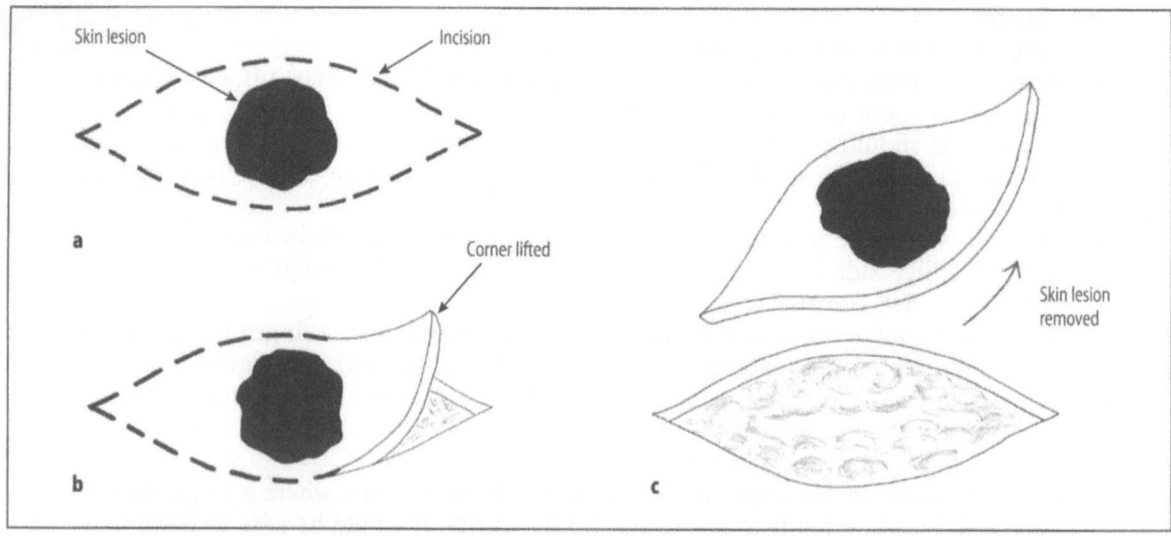

Figure 5.5. a Elliptical incision ... b with corner "lifted" ... c with incision deepened and with lesion dissected off

- Now pull the free corner up and away from the skin using the toothed forceps and deepen the incision along one side of the ellipse using the scalpel. The incision should be made deep enough so that the edges of the wound are separated by a few millimetres. (You may need to move the toothed forceps along the incision as you progress.) See Figure 5.5.
- Continue doing this until the opposite corner has been reached.
- Return to the freed corner and dissect along the other side of the ellipse.
- Free the opposite corner.
- Now grasp one end of the ellipse with the toothed forceps (or you can use a tissue forceps such as an Allis).
- Pull the lesion up and use a scalpel to excise the ellipse of skin from the underlying fat. See Figure 5.5.
- Send the lesion for histology.
- Close the wound with everting sutures (non-absorbable) or subcuticular suture.
- Remove the sutures at the appropriate interval (see Section 2.3).

An alternative to surgical excision is curettage, which is suitable for small lesions. This is done under local anaesthetic. The base of the lesion is scraped out with a curette and allowed to heal. Sutures are not required. Do not forget to send the lesion for histological examination.

5.8 Keloid Scar

A keloid scar is essentially excess growth of scar tissue beyond the extent of the incision or wound margins (in contrast to a hypertrophic scar, which is excess scar tissue within the confines of the incision/wound margins). It is more common in black and dark-skinned people. It may be rather unsightly or cause irritation such as itching, and furthermore may be subject to repeated trauma if in an awkward position. Even if excised, there is a high risk of recurrent keloid formation. Recurrent keloid scarring may be reduced by injection of long-acting steroids into the skin and subcutaneous tissue following excision. Radiotherapy is also sometimes used to avoid recurrence.

Always warn the patient of the possibility of recurrence before undertaking this procedure.

Objective	To excise the scar and form a new neat scar.
Indications	Cosmetic.
	Repeated trauma due to position.
Setting	Operating theatre.
Anaesthetic	Local, or general for larger wounds.
Position	Position the patient to maximise exposure of the area. Ensure that the patient is comfortable.
Preparation	Chlorhexidine (iodine may obscure the scar margins) – use a tissue marker to mark out the edges before preparation if necessary.

Procedure

- Make an elliptical incision around the keloid scar. If possible, use skin creases or Langer's lines.
- Excise the entire scar down to subcutaneous fat using the same technique described for excision of pigmented naevi in Section 5.7.
- Close the wound with a subcuticular suture or adhesive strips if possible.
- Advise the patient to avoid getting the scar wet.
- Remove the suture early (3 to 4 days) and apply adhesive strips to avoid the scar opening up.

5.9 Abscess

An abscess is a collection of pus and usually requires incision and drainage. It can occur in any part of the body but the common areas include the base of the fingernails (paronychia), peri-anal area and breast. Fluctuation and "pointing" of the abscess indicates suitability for drainage. Large abscess cavities often have loculations that must also be broken down.

Objective	To drain the collection of pus.
Indication	To cure the abscess and relieve pain and infection.
Setting	Aseptic conditions for small abscesses that only require lancing.
	Theatre/sterile conditions for larger collections.
Preparation	Cleanse the skin with iodine all over the abscess and surrounding area.
Anaesthetic	Local anaesthesia can be used to lance a small abscess, but it is often difficult to achieve and therefore the procedure can be painful. General anaesthetic allows better drainage.

Position Ensure good exposure. For peri-anal abscesses the lithotomy position is ideal.

Procedure

- In the case of a peri-anal abscess, digital rectal examination, proctoscopy and sigmoidoscopy should be done in order to determine if you are also dealing with a fistula-in-ano.
- It is important that an abscess is drained adequately and that the cavity heals from the deep aspect, rather than the skin healing over the cavity, which may result in recurrence of the abscess. Therefore, most abscesses are dealt with using a cruciate incision or elliptical incision to allow for healing by secondary intention. Small abscesses may sometime be treated by linear incisions.
- If the abscess is small, use a scalpel to make an incision through the skin and into the abscess cavity, placing the incision longitudinally over the summit of the abscess. Pus will extrude immediately and, if under a considerable amount of pressure, may squirt out forcefully.
- For larger abscesses, and in particular a peri-anal abscess, a cruciate incision or elliptical incision is made to ensure the cavity remains open. The skin should be sent for histology if there is the possibility of systemic pathology such as Crohn's disease.
- For a breast abscess, circumferential incisions are cosmetically better.
- Send off a swab for microscopy, culture and sensitivity. If there is a lot of pus, use a syringe to aspirate some and then put the pus in a specimen "pot" to send off for bacteriology.
- Allow the pus to drain. Empty the abscess cavity with finger pressure.
- Insert a finger into the abscess cavity and break down all loculations with a sweeping motion along the inner walls.
- Use a curette to scrape the walls clean.
- Wash out the cavity with normal saline using a syringe.
- Do not close the skin but rather pack the cavity with something suitable such as ribbon gauze soaked in proflavine, leaving the tail end visible.
- Cover with dry dressing gauze and a pad.

Post-op. Change the dressing after 24 hours. The cavity needs to be dressed and repacked regularly, reducing the amount of packing gradually so that it heals from inside outwards.

5.10 Skin Cancers

5.10.1 *Basal Cell Carcinoma*

Also known as "rodent ulcer".

Basal cell carcinoma occurs most commonly on sun-exposed areas, particularly the face. It is classically described as a lesion with a central ulcer with pearly raised edges and telangectasia. It is usually treated by excisional biopsy, but radiotherapy can be used for large lesions or those in awkward positions. Radiotherapy should not be used for lesions in very close proximity to cartilage or bone.

Objective	To excise the entire lesion.
Indication	To "cure" the malignancy, thereby preventing local invasion.
Setting	Operating theatre.
Anaesthetic	Local.
Preparation	Chlorhexidine or povidone-iodine.
Position	Position the patient to maximise exposure of the area. Ensure that the patient is comfortable.

Procedure

- Proceed as for pigmented naevi, using an elliptical incision and ensuring that a clear margin of normal skin of at least 1 mm is obtained.

Post-op.	Remove sutures as appropriate (see section 2.3.7). Review the histology when it is available. If the histology shows incomplete excision but the wound appears to be completely healed with no lesion seen; it is reasonable to review the patient at regular intervals for a few years rather than do a re-excision. If the lesion recurs during review, then a re-excision is necessary; however, if it does not then the patient can be discharged.

5.10.2 Squamous Cell Carcinoma

These lesions can be excised in much the same way as basal cell carcinoma. However, they tend to metastasise, and therefore a clear margin of at least 2 mm should be aimed for (more for large lesions). If histology shows incomplete excision, we recommend re-excision.

5.10.3 Malignant Melanoma

Malignant melanoma is a tumour derived from melanocytes and is highly malignant. The incidence is increasing. The lesions tend to occur on sun-exposed areas. The most common sites are the limbs, including the soles of the feet and palms, and the head and neck. They occasionally occur in the nail bed, i.e. subungual melanoma.

Table 5.1. Malignant melanoma: depth of invasion, and prognosis

Clark's level	Breslow thickness (mm)	Risk
I epidermal	< 0.76	low
II papillary dermis		
III papillary/reticular dermis	0.76 to 1.5	moderate
IV reticular dermis	> 1.5	high
V subcutaneous fat		

Clark, W.A., Jr., From L., Bernardino, E.A., Mitini, M.C.: The histogenesis and biologic behaviour of primary human malignant melanomas of the skin. *Cancer Res*, 29: 705, 1969
Breslow, A: Thickness, cross-sectional areas and depth of invasion in the prognosis of cutaneous melanoma. *Ann. Surgery*, 179: 902, 1970

Table 5.2. Suggested margins of excision of malignant melanoma

Depth of lesion (mm)	Margin (cm)
< 0.76	1
0.76 to 1	2
> 1	3

Most lesions are pigmented. The malignant tendency and hence prognosis depends on the depth of invasion. This has been described by Clark et al. in relation to skin structure, and by Breslow in terms of depth of invasion (see Table 5.1).

Surgical excision is the treatment of choice and must include the full thickness of skin.

In general, the required margin of excision is as shown in Table 5.2.

If a lesion is thought to be a malignant melanoma, it is best to refer the patient to a specialist from the onset.

Objective   To determine whether a lesion is malignant and then treat as necessary.
                  To excise the lesion completely.
Indications   Skin lesion suspicious of malignancy.
                  For small lesions, excision biopsy is carried out.
                  For large lesions, incision biopsy is required to confirm the diagnosis first.
                  If malignancy is confirmed, then a wider excision will be required and the patient should be referred to a specialist for treatment. In some cases, nodal excision will also be required.
Setting   Operating theatre/sterile conditions.
Position   Expose the area adequately.
Preparation   Cleanse the skin with iodine solution, or chlorhexidine if the margins would be obscured.
Anaesthetic   Local anaesthetic is adequate for small well-demarcated lesions. General anaesthesia is required for wider excision.

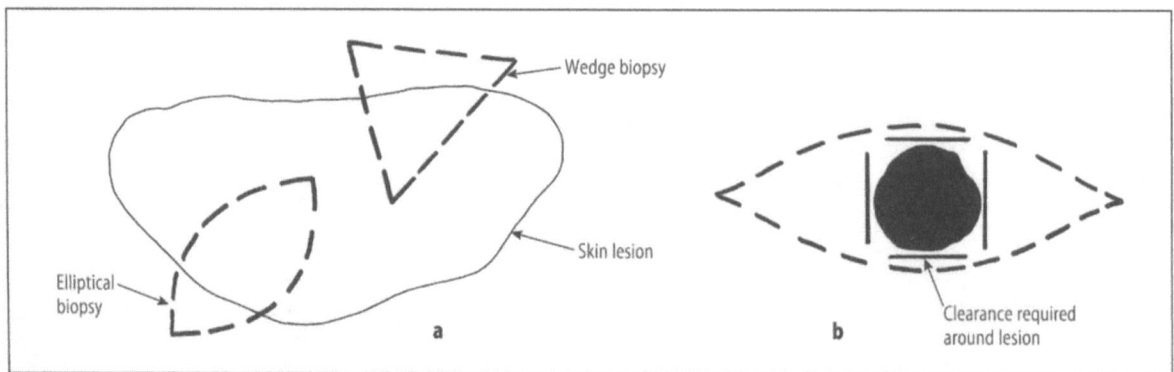

Figure 5.6. Incisional biopsy of a suspected melanoma (a), excisional biopsy (b)

Procedure

- Incision biopsy – a wedge of the lesion will suffice. Alternatively, an elliptical skin biopsy can be taken. Make clean neat incisions with a scalpel. Send off for histology. See Figure 5.6a.
- Excision biopsy – Make an elliptical incision around the lesion with a 5mm margin (see Figure 5.6b). Use a skin crease if possible and proceed as for excision of pigmented naevi.

Post-op.   Remove the sutures as appropriate (see section 2.3.7).

Check on the histology and refer to hospital if necessary.

5.11 Pinch Skin Graft

Pinch grafts are used to cover areas of skin loss. A donor site is required, such as the thigh, from which small pieces of skin are taken and then placed over the area to be covered. For best results the ulcerated area should not be grossly infected and should have healthy granulation tissue visible. Colonisation with aggressive organisms reduces the chances of success. Taking a culture swab before the procedure and treating any aggressive organisms will increase the chances of the graft "taking".

Objective	To attain skin cover and aid the healing of an ulcerated area of the skin.
Indication	An open wound, which is too large to heal well without additional skin cover, for example venous ulceration or traumatic ulceration. Large areas of ulceration may take a long time to heal and are at risk of infection.
Setting	Operating theatre/sterile conditions.
Position	Expose both areas adequately (donor and recipient).
Anaesthetic	Local.
	Infiltrate the skin and subcutaneous tissue of the donor areas generously.
	If a large number of pinch grafts are needed, general anaesthetic may be more suitable.

Procedure

- Cleanse both areas of skin with iodine.
- Use fine forceps to tent up the skin. Excise small pieces of skin. See Figure 5.7.
- Cover the donor area temporarily with a wet swab.
- Place the excised pieces of skin over the recipient wound. See Figure 5.7.
- The graft can be secured with a suture or a staple but we do not recommend this.
- Cover the wound with paraffin gauze and a dry dressing.
- Keep area immobilised for 10 days.
- Remove dressing carefully (they may need to be soaked off).

Note: if a large number of pinch grafts are needed, it is also possible to excise an ellipse of skin (one piece sufficient to supply all the pinch grafts) from the donor area and

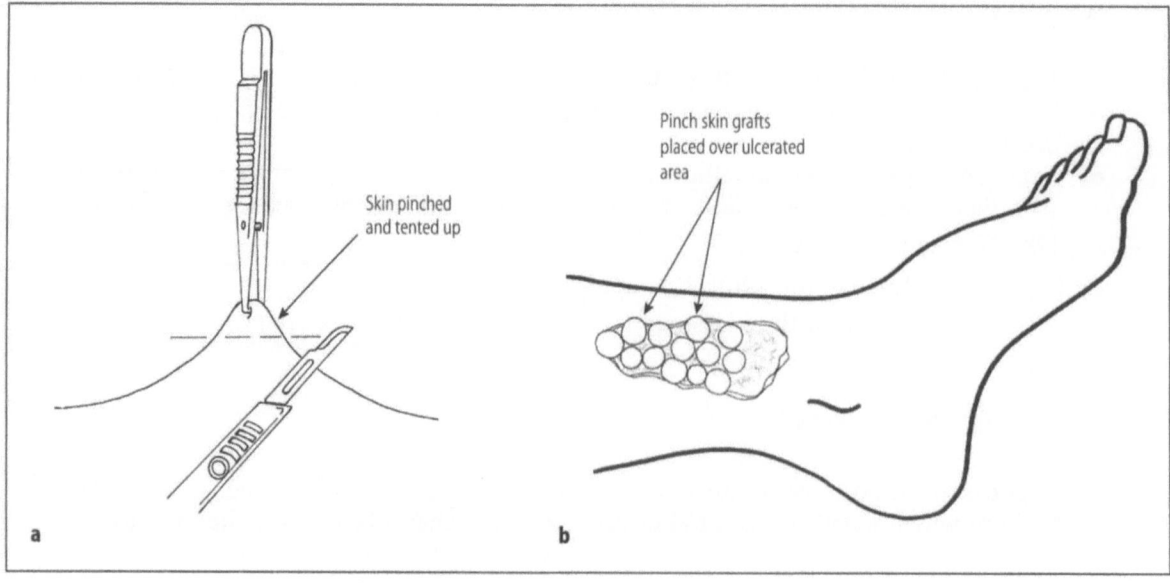

Figure 5.7. **a** Harvesting of graft . . . **b** graft applied to ulcer

close the wound primarily. Then cut up the removed piece into small pieces and apply it onto the recipient area as described above.

5.12 Warts and Verrucas

These are caused by a viral infection and can occur anywhere on the body.

Peri-anal warts are dealt with in Chapter 8. Verrucas are commonly seen on the soles of the feet and are associated with hyperkeratinisation.

Non-surgical treatment options include:

- salicylic acid application
- freezing with nitrous oxide-cryosurgery
- application of podophyllin.

Surgical options are curetting and excision.

Curetting
This is usually only suitable for small lesions.

Procedure

- Clean the skin with antiseptic solution.
- Infiltrate the skin with local anaesthetic.
- Curette the wart from the skin until bleeding occurs.

- Diathermy may be required for haemostasis.
- Cover with a dry dressing.

Excision
This is usually performed for large warts or recurrent lesions.

Procedure

- Clean the skin with antiseptic solution.
- Infiltrate the skin with local anaesthetic.
- Make an elliptical incision around the wart.
- Remove the ellipse of skin, as described for pigmented naevi, Section 5.7.
- Send for histology.
- Close the wound with interrupted sutures.
- Apply a dry dressing.
- Remove the sutures after 7 days.

5.13 Skin Biopsy

A skin biopsy is performed to make a histological diagnosis; for example:

- where a large pigmented lesion is suspected to be malignant melanoma but extensive surgery would be required to ensure adequate removal
- to detect malignant change in a long-standing ulcer – Marjolin's ulcer
- to determine the nature of a skin condition such as vasculitis.

Objective	To obtain a representative skin sample for a histological diagnosis. The sample of skin should include the area affected and the adjacent normal skin.
Indication	Suspected pathology.
Setting	Aseptic technique or operating theatre.
Position	Ensure good exposure.
Anaesthetic	Local.

Procedure

- Make an elliptical incision to encompass the edge of the skin lesion and the adjacent healthy tissue.
- Excise the ellipse with the full thickness of skin.
- Send for histology.
- Close the wound with interrupted 3/0 Prolene sutures.
- Remove sutures after 7 days.
- If it is not possible to appose the skin edges, cover the defect with paraffin gauze and a dry dressing.

5.14 Other Lesions

5.14.1 Solar Keratosis

These are found on sun exposed areas of the body, often seen on the back of the hand. They can be excised in the same way as pigmented naevi (see Section 5.7) or they can be "shaved" off with a scalpel.

5.14.2 Seborrheic Wart

These are common in the elderly, increasing in incidence with age. A seborrheic wart is a raised dark lesion that looks like a plaque that could be peeled off the skin. It is often seen on the trunk. It can be "shaved" off the skin with a scalpel or excised in the same way as a naevus (see Section 5.7). If there is any suspicion that the lesion is a basal cell carcinoma (BCC) then it should be excised fully as described in Section 5.10.1.

5.14.3 Bowen's Disease

This is an epithelial lesion that represents carcinoma-in-situ. It may progress to squamous cell carcinoma. Surgical excision is diagnostic as well as therapeutic and should be done in the same way as pigmented naevi (see Section 5.7).

5.14.4 Miscellaneous Skin Lesions

There are numerous other minor skin lesions that occur with varying frequency. These can usually be excised in the same way as pigmented naevi (see Section 5.7) and should always be sent for histology.

6 Varicose Veins

6.1 Introduction

Varicose veins result from a failure of valves in the superficial venous system (long or short saphenous systems), and the condition is usually associated with incompetence (or reflux) in one of the main junctions between the superficial and deep systems, namely the sapheno-femoral junction or the sapheno-popliteal junction. Less commonly reflux is from incompetent perforators such as the mid-thigh perforator or others. Varicose veins may be "primary" due to damaged valves, or "secondary" due to deep venous incompetence.

Varicose vein surgery is ideally suited for day-case surgery. However, we believe that for day-case surgery to be safe, only one leg should be operated on and the patient not turned (as is required if both the sapheno-femoral and sapheno-popliteal junctions are incompetent) during the operation. Doing more than that prolongs the operative time and subsequent recovery time, and makes planning and running of lists more difficult.

6.2 Indications for Surgery

Varicose vein surgery is indicated for symptomatic veins (aching, swelling, throbbing and other non-specific symptoms), for cosmetic reasons and for effecting the healing (or prevention of recurrence) of venous ulcers due to superficial venous disease. To ensure that the correct procedure is performed and the best result obtained, the patient needs to be investigated to delineate the site(s) of incompetence causing the varicosities.

6.3 Investigations

Clinical examination alone is inaccurate in determining the site(s) of reflux, especially in complicated cases. Hand-held Doppler in experienced hands give accurate results in the groin, but is less accurate in the popliteal fossa. Furthermore, the accuracy diminishes further in the case of recurrent varicose veins, or mixed superficial and deep venous incompetence. Duplex scanning (B-mode ultrasound combined with pulsed Doppler sonography and colour flow mapping) is the current gold standard in the investigation of the venous system and accurately determines which veins and junctions are incompetent. Radiological studies such as varicography and phlebography are invasive and seldom performed except, perhaps, on-table venography for determining the sapheno-popliteal junction (see below).

6.4 Treatment Rationale

The site(s) of incompetence must be determined. Duplex scanning or hand-held Doppler studies best do this. Duplex scanning will also determine the state of the deep veins. If there is any suspicion that the deep venous system is occluded, then varicose vein surgery must *not* be undertaken, and referral to a specialist unit is advised. The recommended treatment for the common patterns of incompetence is discussed below.

6.4.1 Sapheno-femoral Junction Incompetence with Long Saphenous Varices

This is the commonest pattern of incompetence found. The recommended treatment for this is sapheno-femoral junction flush ligation, stripping of the long saphenous vein to the upper calf, and avulsion of varicosities through small cosmetic skin incisions.

Causes of Failure and Pitfalls
Failure to strip the long saphenous vein results in increased incidence of recurrence, either due to reconnection of the long saphenous vein with the femoral vein (missed tributaries or angioneogenesis), or due to incompetence of a mid-thigh perforator.

Stripping too far down (in the past the vein was stripped from groin to ankle) results in an unacceptable rate of damage to the saphenous nerve. This is intimately related to the long saphenous vein from about the junction of the middle calf with the upper calf down to the ankle. Failure to appreciate the presence of a duplex long saphenous system (seen in some patients) may result in failure to strip the haemodynamically important incompetent vein; this can be avoided by careful pre-operative assessment.

Ligation, stripping of the wrong vein (i.e. femoral) or indeed an artery (stripping of the superficial femoral artery has been reported) should not occur if the recommended operative technique is followed. If either does occur, and this is recognised at operation, a vascular surgeon should be called immediately to assess the situation.

6.4.2 Sapheno-popliteal Junction Incompetence with Short Saphenous Varices

The recommended treatment for this is sapheno-popliteal junction ligation, and avulsion of varicosities through small cosmetic skin incisions. Stripping of the short saphenous vein is carried out by some surgeons and probably reduces the incidence of recurrence. However, this may cause damage to the sural nerve, which has a very intimate relationship with this vein. "Inversion" stripping, as opposed to conventional stripping (see Section 6.8), may avoid this problem.

Causes of Failure and Pitfalls
The main cause of failure of this operation is poor pre-operative marking. This is because the sapheno-popliteal junction may be anywhere between 10 cm below and 10 cm above the popliteal skin crease. To avoid this, the proximal part of the short saphenous vein and the sapheno-popliteal junction should be marked pre-operatively using a permanent

(non-water-soluble) marker. Careless dissection in the popliteal fossa may also result in damage to the tibial nerve, popliteal vein and popliteal artery.

6.4.3 Combined Sapheno-femoral and Sapheno-popliteal Junction Incompetence with Long and Short Saphenous Varices

In this case both junctions need to be tackled. On a day-case basis we only recommend one system to be done at a time. This is because doing both prolongs the operation and anaesthetic time, as well as necessitating the turning of the patient during the operation.

6.4.4 Varicosities with no Junction Incompetence

In these cases sclerotherapy or avulsions through small skin incisions is sufficient to effect treatment. Avulsions may be undertaken under local or general anaesthetic, depending on the number to be performed.

6.4.5 Calf Perforator Incompetence

Varicose veins solely as a result of calf perforator incompetence (without sapheno-femoral or sapheno-popliteal junction incompetence) are not common. Usually, avulsion of the varicosities through small skin incisions is sufficient to achieve good results. However, some surgeons believe that this is inadequate, in which case pre-operative marking and tying of the perforators is performed.

6.5 Recurrent Varicose Veins

The rationale in these cases is no different to that discussed above. The site(s) of incompetence should be delineated and tackled. In the case of recurrence due to a mid-thigh perforator in an unstripped long saphenous vein, the recommended treatment is stripping of the long saphenous vein from its highest point to the upper calf. Recurrent varicose vein surgery (with the exception of multiple avulsions only) is a difficult procedure and should only be undertaken by those familiar with it.

6.6 Sclerotherapy

Equipment needed:

Syringes	Disposable 1 ml or 2 ml syringes.
Needles	Disposable 20G, 25G or 27G.
Compression pads	These are placed on the sclerosed veins for compression and can be cut to size. They may be made from rubber or cotton (dental rolls are often used for this purpose).
Bandages	Stretch bandages such as crepe bandage.

Adhesive tape	Such as 1-inch micropore.
Sclerosant	Such as sodium tetradecyl sulphate 1 per cent solution.

Sclerotheraphy Technique

A number of techniques for sclerotherapy have been described. The one described below is based on the Fegan method.

Objective	To sclerose varicose veins.
Indications	Patients with minor varicosities or reticular veins for symptomatic or cosmetic reasons. Duplex scanning should be first undertaken to ensure that there is no major junction incompetence.
Setting	Outpatient department using aseptic technique.
Position	On examination couch (see below).
Anaesthetic	None.

Preparation

- The sites of the varicosities to be injected are determined and marked with a suitable skin marker. This is best done with the patient standing, since the varicosities will be most obvious in this position.
- The patient is then asked to sit upright on a couch with the leg horizontal. In this position the vein should be full enough to make venepuncture possible.
- If not, the leg can be dangled down on the edge of the couch.

Injection Technique

- A 2 ml syringe is used with a suitable needle (the smaller the vein, the smaller the needle needed).
- Draw up 1 ml of sclerosant solution (use higher concentrations for large veins and lower concentrations for small veins).
- Insert the needle into the pre-marked varicosity with the leg in the horizontal or dependant position (see above).
- Aspirate a little blood to ensure that you are in the vein.
- Hold the syringe firmly against the leg to avoid the needle moving position and ask the patient to lie back and raise the leg up to empty the vein.
- Compress the vein to be injected on either side of the needle using two fingers (your fingers should be about 3 cm apart).
- Inject 0.5 to 1 ml of the sclerosant into the vein. This should be painless. If the patient feels stinging, this indicates that sclerosant is being injected subcutaneously. Stop injecting and start the process again.
- Remove the needle but keep your fingers compressing the vein for 30 s.
- The most distal varicosity is injected first followed by the next most distal varicosity and so on.
- As each varicosity is injected, a compression pad is applied to the site and compressed by wrapping the limb up to that point with a crepe bandage.
- If two sites are at about the same level on the leg they cannot both be injected at the same session.

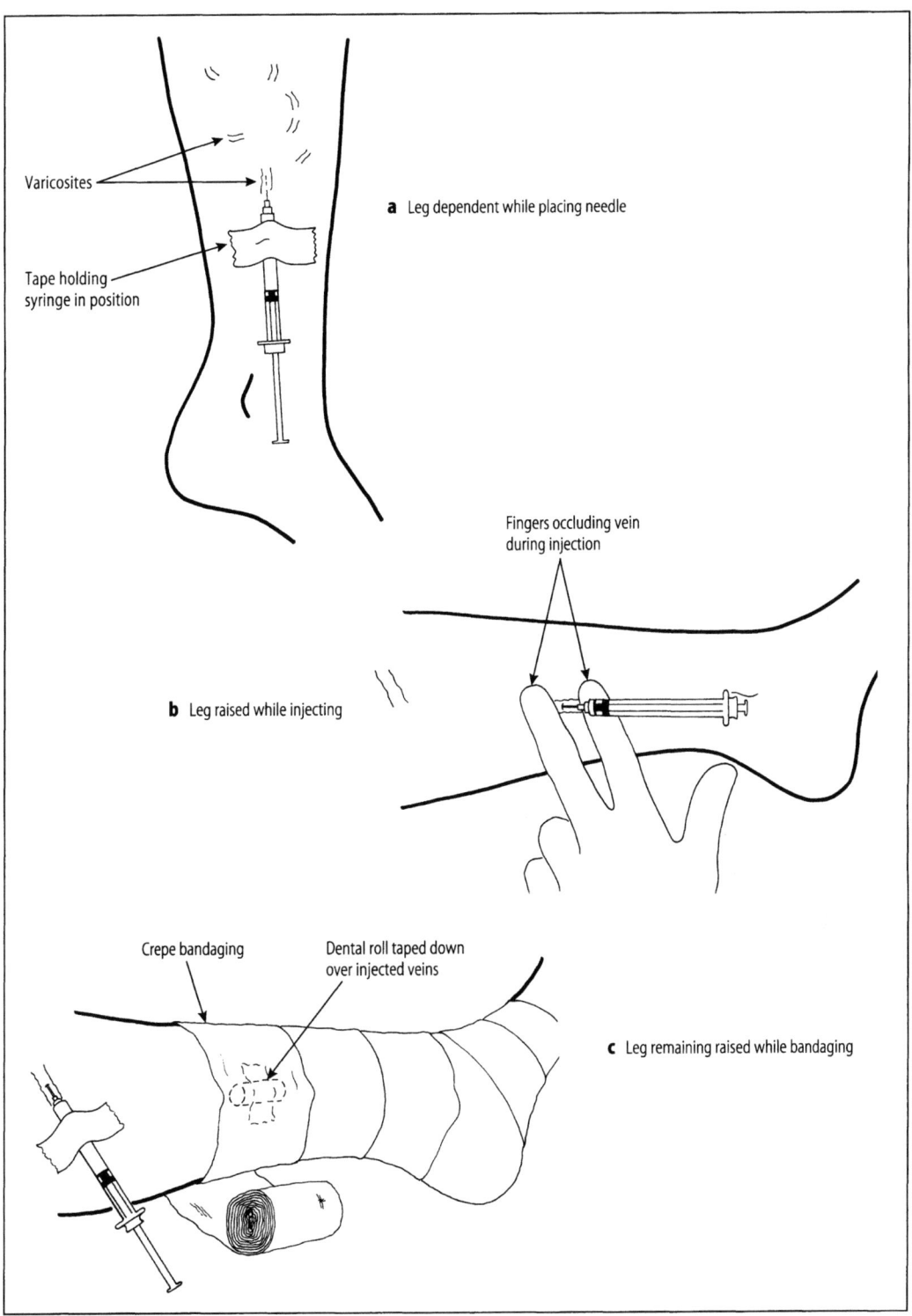

Figure 6.1. Injection sclerotherapy

- Apply a compression stocking on top of the bandages.
- See the patient in 1 to 2 weeks to check the result. The patient will need to wear compression stockings for 3 to 6 weeks (opinion about this varies; we recommend 4 weeks).

6.7 Junction Ligation

6.7.1 Sapheno-femoral Junction

This operation may be done under local or general anaesthetic. Our practice is to do it under general anaesthetic, as we believe that not combining it with stripping of the long saphenous vein results in an increased risk of recurrence. We also perform phlebectomies of the varicosities at the same time. However, some surgeons perform sapheno-femoral ligation under local anaesthetic, no stripping of the long saphenous vein and injection sclerotherapy of the varicosities as an outpatient at a later date.

Objective	Treatment of varicose veins due to sapheno-femoral junction incompetence.
Indication	Varicose veins due to incompetence of the sapheno-femoral junction.
Setting	Operating theatre.
Position	The patient is placed flat on the back with a head-down tilt sufficient to empty the varicosities and reduce venous pressure and thus bleeding. The legs are abducted, and this can be achieved by the use of a leg board. See Figure 6.2.
Anaesthetic	General.

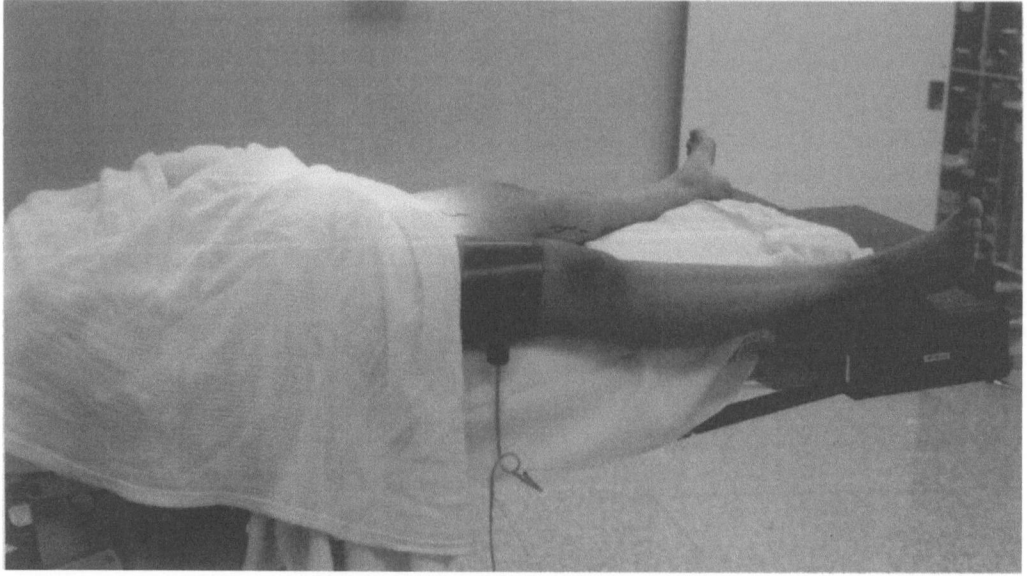

Figure 6.2. Position of patient for varicose vein surgery

Procedure

- Prepare the skin with an antiseptic solution (use an aqueous rather than an alcoholic solution to prevent the pre-operative marking of the varicose veins being rubbed off).
- Towel as appropriate. We use a waterproof towel covered by a large towel (both under the leg) a large towel over the trunk from the groin upwards, two side towels and a glove or small towel to cover the foot. All exposed areas should have been prepared beforehand.
- Get the go-ahead from the anaesthetist to start the operation.
- Palpate for the femoral artery, and map in your mind its position. Remember that it is one finger breadth in diameter, and imagine the femoral vein which is also one finger breadth in diameter lying next to it medially.
- Using a no. 10 blade, make a transverse skin crease incision of about 4 cm in length in the groin crease centred on where you imagine the femoral vein to be.
- Deepen the incision into the subcutaneous fat along the line of the incision.
- The superficial fascia of the thigh will now be encountered. This is a very definite layer that is easy to see.
- Incise the superficial fascia along the line of the skin incision. Ensure that you do not go deep at this point, as often there is only a thin layer of deep fat below the superficial fascia protecting the veins (especially in thin patients).
- Usually there is minimal bleeding in the incision, and diathermy is not needed. However, if bleeding from the edges of the wound obscures the view, achieve haemostasis using unipolar or bipolar diathermy.
- Take a swab (4 × 4 or similar), unfold it, and by pressing it into the wound with the index finger of your right hand, sweep the deep fat of the thigh distally towards the foot. This almost always reveals the long saphenous vein. The same motion can be performed upwards to clear the fat from the area of interest. Some practice is needed to learn what degree of force is required to do this. Too much force and small veins may be torn, resulting in bleeding; too little force and the fat won't be cleared (see Figure 6.3).
- Place a small mastoid self-retaining retractor in the wound with its jaws deep to the superficial fascia, spreading the wound open in an up-down direction. Ask your assistant to place two small Langenbeck retractors in each side of the wound (medial and lateral) and retract. This four-way retraction ensures good exposure of the operative field.
- If the long saphenous vein is not seen by this stage, then (1) ensure that you are in the correct position by palpating for the femoral artery again and ensuring that you are just medial to it, (2) make sure that you are deep to the superficial fascia of the thigh, (3) repeat the process of pushing the fat away, and the long saphenous vein should come into view.
- Pick up the long saphenous vein with a pair of thick non-toothed forceps about 2 cm away from where you think the sapheno-femoral junction is located, and start cleaning it and its tributaries of the fat, which should strip away quite easily. A number of instruments may be used to do this, including another pair of non-toothed forceps, the closed ends of curved non-pointed scissors, or a small swab held in a suitable instrument (Lahey swab). Continue cleaning the long saphenous vein and its tributaries proximally until the sapheno-femoral junction is seen. You

should not cut any veins until this stage. Once you are sure that you have seen the sapheno-femoral junction, you may proceed to the next stage. *You must be satisfied that what you are looking at is the sapheno-femoral junction*, i.e. a superficial vein which has tributaries, is diving down to join a deeper vein, and that you can demonstrate the upward and downward continuation of the deeper vein.

- Apply arterial clips to the tributaries of the long saphenous vein as far away from their confluence as possible.
- Apply another arterial clip to the long saphenous vein distal to where all the tributaries join it.
- Apply a further arterial clip 0.5 cm away from the sapheno-femoral junction (on the long saphenous vein side). This last arterial clip should be cephaloid to where the tributaries join the long saphenous vein.
- Cut the tributaries of the long saphenous vein proximal to the clips.
- Cut the segment of long saphenous vein between the two clips on it.
- Tie all the tributaries with a suitable suture material such as 2/0 Vicryl. Double tie

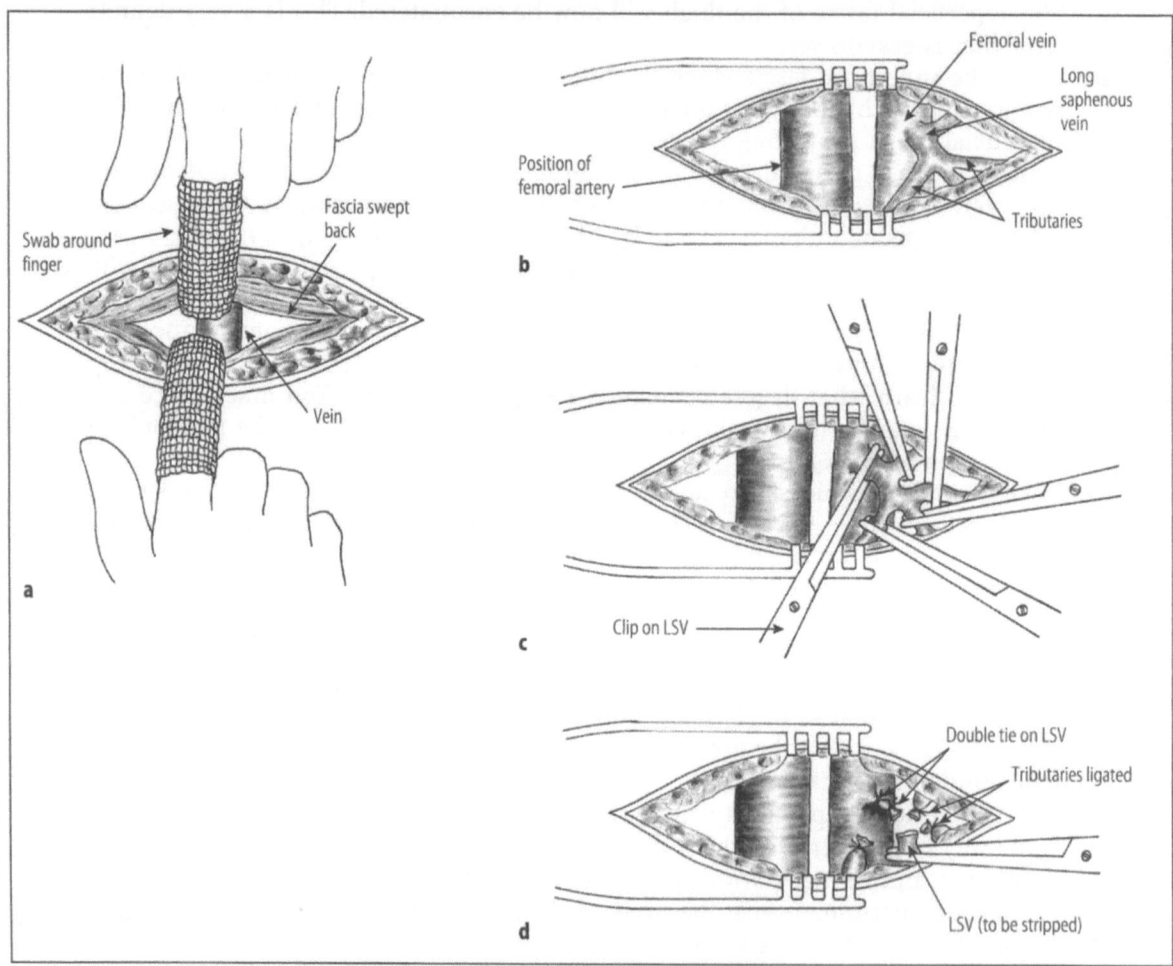

Figure 6.3. Dissection of the sapheno-femoral junction

the sapheno-femoral junction flush with the femoral vein using 0 Vicryl (some surgeons recommend a transfixion stitch). Ensure not to pull on the arterial clip as you are doing this, since this may "tent up" the femoral vein, and the tie may narrow it. Pulling too hard on the arterial clip may also result in avulsing the long saphenous vein off the femoral vein or tearing the junction. If this happens, the femoral vein must be repaired using 5/0 or 6/0 Prolene.

- Check for haemostasis, and achieve this with diathermy if needed.
- The long saphenous vein (which still has a clip applied beyond the cut end) is now ready for stripping. If stripping is not to be performed then tie the long saphenous vein with a suitable material (for example 2/0 Vicryl), otherwise strip the long saphenous vein as described below.
- After ensuring haemostasis, close the superficial fascia of the thigh with interrupted absorbable sutures, such as 2/0 or 3/0 Vicryl or Dexon.
- Inject local anaesthetic (such as 10 ml, 0.5 per cent Bupivicaine) into the wound – ensure the local anaesthetic is not injected into a vessel.
- Close the skin with a subcuticular monofilament suture such as nylon, 3/0 Prolene or PDS.
- Clean and dry the wound and apply a sterile occlusive dressing.

6.7.2 Sapheno-popliteal Junction

The sapheno-popliteal junction is variable in position. It is usually within 2 cm of the popliteal skin crease but may be up to 10 cm above or below it. Therefore, this junction must be marked pre-operatively. This is best done by duplex scanning, but if this is not available then hand-help Doppler is satisfactory. If neither is available, then intra-operative phlebography may be needed (an arterial clip is placed to mark the popliteal skin crease, contrast is injected into the short saphenous vein and an on-table X-ray is taken).

The operation may be done under local or general anaesthetic. Our practice is to do it under general anaesthetic, as it is an uncomfortable position for the patient. This also enables us to perform phlebectomies of the varicosities at the same time.

Objective	To treat varicose veins due to sapheno-popliteal junction incompetence.
Indications	Sapheno-popliteal junction incompetence.
Setting	Operating theatre.
Position	The patient is placed prone (on the front) with a head-down tilt sufficient to empty the varicosities and reduce venous pressure and thus bleeding. The chest and pelvis are supported on pillows and the arms placed above the head.
Anaesthetic	General.

Procedure

- Prepare the skin with an antiseptic solution (use an aqueous rather than an alcoholic solution to prevent the pre-operative marking of the varicose veins being rubbed off).
- Towel as appropriate. We use a waterproof towel covered by a large towel under the leg, a large towel from the mid-thigh upwards, two side towels and a medium

towel to cover the lower third of the calf and foot. All exposed areas should have been prepared beforehand.
- Get the go-ahead from the anaesthetist to start the operation.
- Make a transverse skin incision 3 cm long and about 1 to 2 cm below the marked sapheno-popliteal junction (see Figure 6.4).
- The incision is made lower than the sapheno-popliteal junction, because at its proximal end the short saphenous vein dives deep, and it is easier to find it before it does this. Once identified, it can be followed to the sapheno-popliteal junction.
- Deepen the skin incision through the subcutaneonus fat and the superficial fascia of the popliteal fossa, and sweep the fat away as described in Section 6.7.1. The short saphenous vein will now become visible.
- Pick up the short saphenous vein with a pair of non-toothed forceps and dissect the fat away from it. Be careful of damage to the tibial nerve, which is in close proximity. Therefore, stay close to the vein during the dissection.
- Follow the vein proximally until you find its junction with the popliteal vein.
- Apply two arterial clips onto the short saphenous vein, one just distal to the sapheno-popliteal junction, and the other a few centimetres further distally.
- Excise the segment of short saphenous vein between the two clips and tie the ends with a suitable material such as 0 Vicryl if no stripping of the short saphenous vein is to be done, otherwise only tie the proximal end (some surgeons recommend a transfixion stitch).
- Stripping of the short saphenous vein can now be undertaken (if required) as described in Section 6.8.
- Check for any bleeding and, if there is any, stop it using diathermy.
- Close the fascia with interrupted sutures using an absorbable material such as 2/0 Vicryl or Dexon.

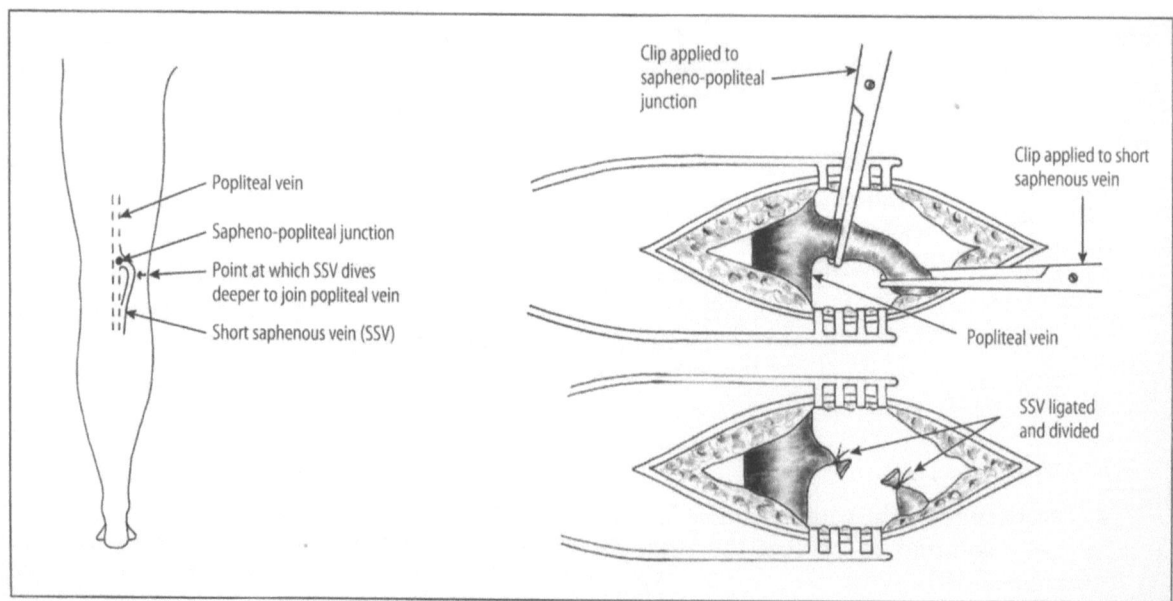

Figure 6.4. Dissection of the sapheno-popliteal junction

- Inject local anaesthetic (such as 10 ml, 0.5 per cent Bupivicaine) into the wound – ensure you do not inject into a vessel).
- Close the skin with a subcuticular monofilament suture such as 3/0 Prolene or PDS.
- Perform multiple phlebectomies as described in Section 6.9.
- Clean and dry the wound and apply a sterile occlusive dressing.

6.8 Stripping

Both the long saphenous and short saphenous veins may be stripped. We recommend stripping the long saphenous vein from groin to the upper calf. Stripping beyond this may cause damage to the saphenous nerve. Not stripping the long saphenous vein is associated with an increased risk of recurrence.

We selectively strip the short saphenous vein down to mid-calf using the inversion method, as this is less likely to cause damage to the sural nerve. We only strip this vein if it is grossly incompetent and dilated.

The techniques for stripping described below are identical for the long saphenous vein and short saphenous vein.

Objective	Stripping of the long saphenous vein or short saphenous vein, usually in conjunction with sapheno-femoral junction or sapheno-popliteal junction incompetence, respectively.
Indications	Long saphenous vein/short saphenous vein incompetence.
Setting	Operating theatre.
Position	Supine for long saphenous vein, prone for short saphenous vein, both with Trendelenburg tilt.
Anaesthetic	General.

6.8.1 Conventional Stripping

Procedure: method 1

- Either a reusable or disposable stripper may be used.
- Apply two arterial clips (use mosquito clips) to opposite walls of the vein to be stripped.
- Loosely place a tie around the long saphenous vein beyond the clips using 0 Vicryl.
- Introduce the stripper into the lumen of the vein and now tighten the previously applied loose tie to stop back-bleeding from the vein.
- Advance the stripper down the vein to the required level – to the upper calf in the case of the long saphenous vein and to mid-calf in the case of the short saphenous vein; see Figure 6.5.
- If there is difficulty in passing the stripper down due to tortuosity of the vein, twist the stripper in either direction, and in the case of the long saphenous vein, try bending the knee slightly. Usually with these manoeuvres the stripper will pass down. Very occasionally it will get stuck just above the knee, and in those circumstances, stripping to that point only can be performed.
- The position of the lower end of the stripper can be determined by palpation.

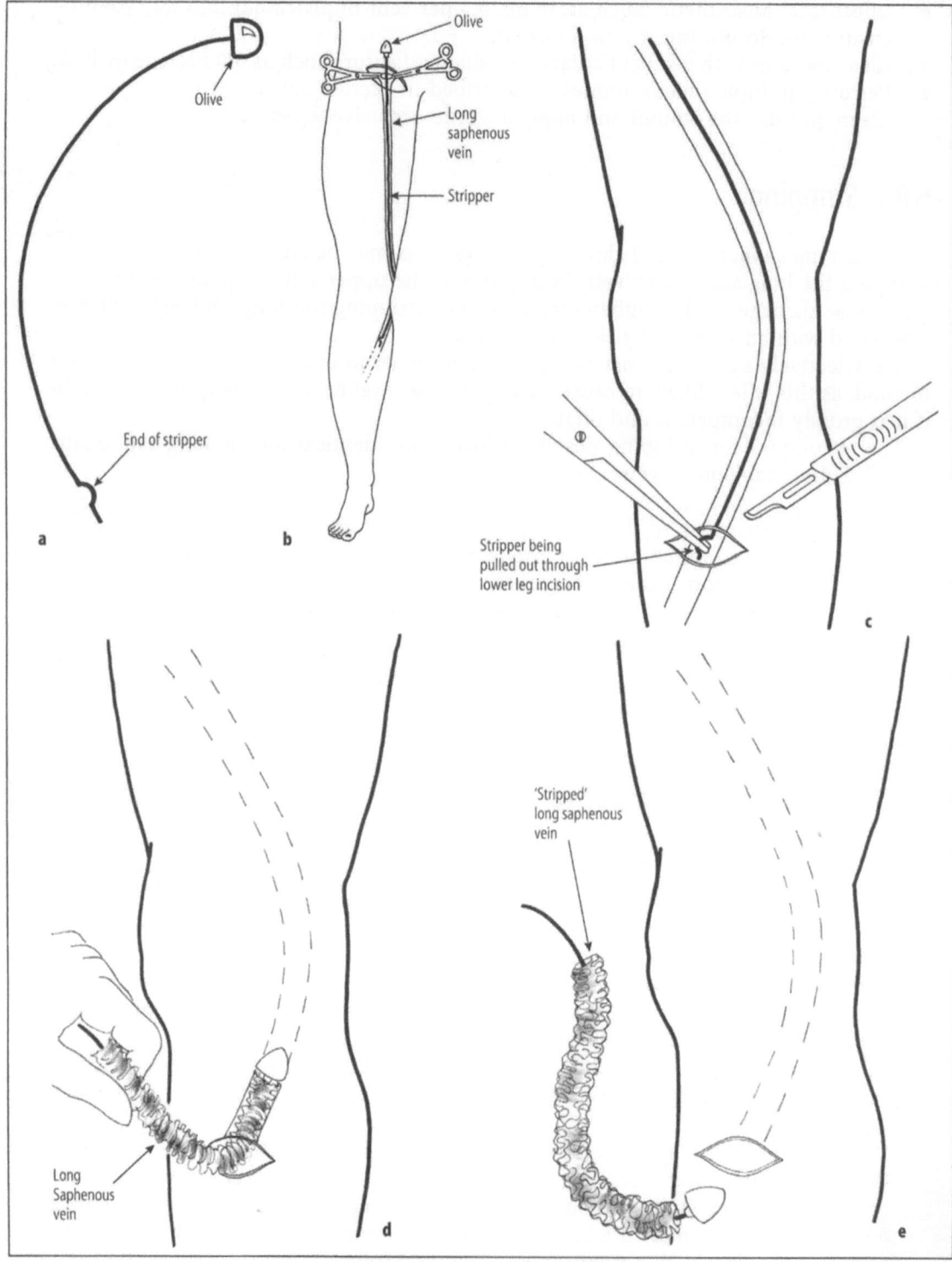

Figure 6.5. Vein stripping – method 1

- When the lower end of the stripper is at the required position, make a stab incision (2 to 3 mm in length) in the skin overlying the lower end of the stripper.
- Put an arterial clip (use mosquito clip) with the jaws open into the incision and grab the vein and the stripper within it and pull them out of the wound. During this manoeuvre the end of the stripper will pierce the wall of the vein and come out of the vein.
- Push the top end of the stripper down until it is near the top end of the wound.
- Engage the olive (the medium size is adequate for most veins) onto the stripper.
- Pull the distal end of the stripper until the olive has reached the lower incision.
- Enlarge the lower skin incision sufficiently to be able to pull the olive and the stripped vein out.
- If the vein distal to the skin incision is still attached to the proximal end, avulse as much of it as possible.
- Close the skin incision with a suitable monofilament subcuticular suture such as 3/0 Prolene or PDS.

Procedure: method 2
This method has the advantage of producing a much smaller distal incision and is our preferred method of stripping. The first steps of the operation are the same as above (until the olive is engaged onto the top end of the stripper).

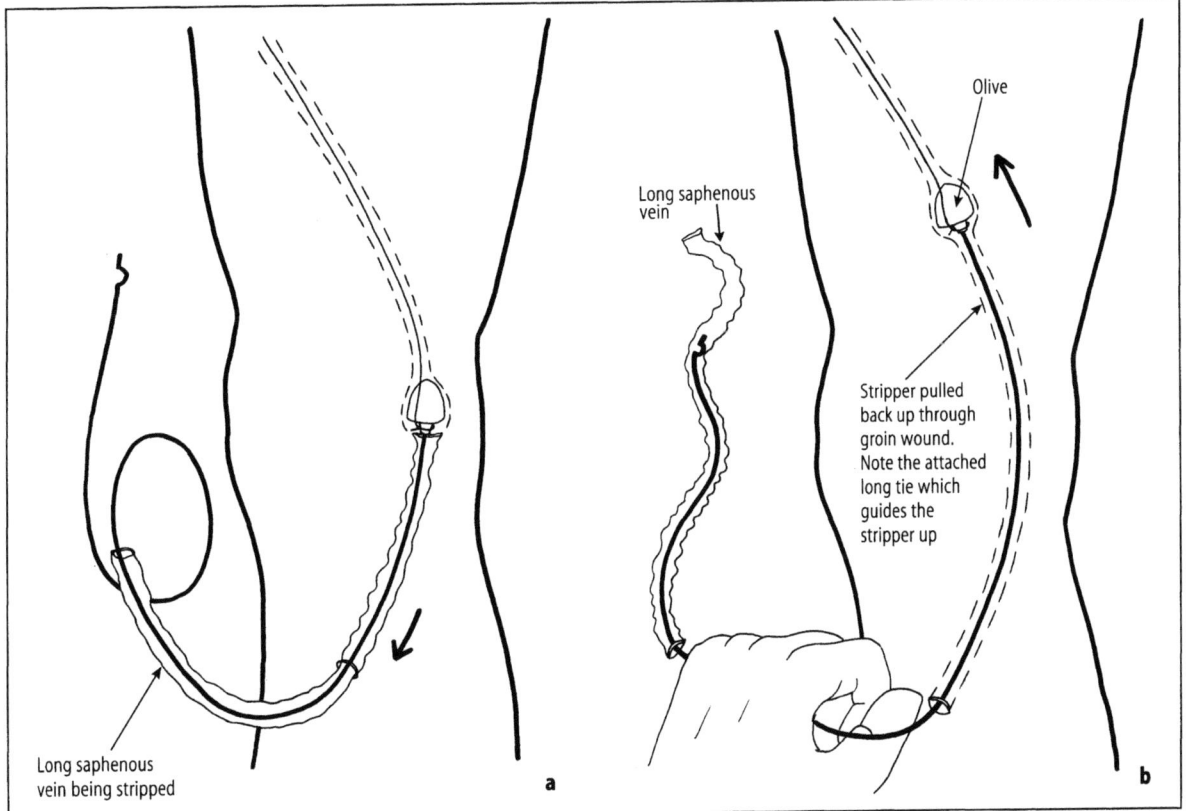

Figure 6.6. Vein stripping – method 2

- Perform the first ten steps described in method 1.
- Tie a strong long tie (such as 0 Vicryl) onto the olive (this can only be done with the disposable stripper since it is grooved). The tie needs to be longer than the distance between the top (groin) and bottom (calf) incisions.
- Pull the distal end of the stripper down while an assistant gently holds the tie at the top end, keeping it very slightly under tension.
- When the olive has reached the bottom wound, place an arterial clip into the bottom wound and grab the vein that is compressed onto the stripper. Pull the full length of the stripped vein out of the wound. It is often easier to pull the vein out when the stripper is eased back (cranoid) slightly.
- Ask the assistant to pull the suture tied onto the olive in a steady manner, while you feed the stripper upwards as it is pulled up.
- When the olive reaches the top wound, ask the assistant to pick it up and pull it and the stripper out.
- The lower incision, which has not needed to be extended (compared to method 1), does not need suturing and can be treated in the same manner as a multiple phlebectomy incision (see Section 6.9).

6.8.2 Inversion Stripping

In this technique the vein is turned inside out as it is being stripped. This makes it less likely for adjacent structures, such as nerves, to be damaged. It is particularly useful for stripping the short saphenous vein. We use the pin stripper for this technique (see Figure 6.7).

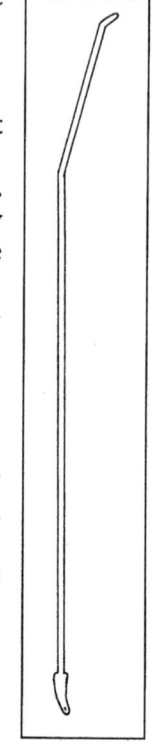

- Apply two arterial clips onto opposite walls of the vein to be stripped.
- Choose the appropriate length of pin stripper needed. They come in three different lengths.
- Insert the angled end of the pin stripper into the lumen of the vein (see Figure 6.7).
- Glide the stripper down the vein, keeping the tip pointing upwards. If there is any difficulty, apply an arterial clip onto the flat proximal end of the stripper and use the clip to turn the pin stripper in either direction to negotiate a tortuous vein.
- Once the distal end of the stripper has reached the correct level, make a stab incision in the skin overlying the end of the stripper using a no. 11 blade.
- Push the end of the stripper out of the vein and out of the skin incision.
- Apply an arterial clip onto the bottom end to avoid it slipping back into the wound.
- Advance the stripper down until the proximal end has come close to the top of the vein.
- Tie a long strong tie (such as 0 Vicryl) onto the end of the stripper, leaving one end 10 cm long and the other the full length of the suture. Ensure that the knot will not slip. Tie a further knot about 3 cm from the end of the stripper.
- Pull the stripper from the distal end until the knot away from the stripper just enters the lumen of the vein.
- Tie the suture around the vein at each arterial clip, ensuring that you have obtained a good grip on the vein with the knot.
- Pull the stripper from the distal end. This should invert the vein onto itself and strip it.
- Keep pulling until the stripper is out, followed by a segment of suture followed by the inverted vein, and followed by the remainder of the suture.

Figure 6.7.
A pin stripper

- If the knot slips off the stripper and only the stripper emerges, the vein can be pulled back using the suture at the top end of the wound, and the process repeated.
- Avulse the distal end of the vein in the distal incision.
- The lower wound is treated in the same manner as a multiple phlebectomy incision (see Section 6.9).

6.9 Avulsion of Varicosities (Phlebectomies)

The veins to be avulsed must be marked pre-operatively using a permanent skin marker, with the patient standing up.

Objective	To remove varicosities.
Indications	Varicose veins with or without junction incompetence.
Setting	Operating theatre.
Position	Supine or prone depending on site (usually with Trendelenburg tilt).
Anaesthetic	Usually general, but local can be used if there are only few varicosities to be avulsed.

Procedure

- Make a stab incision directly over the marked vein of about 2 mm length using a no. 11 blade.
- Using a hook (phlebectomy hook or skin hook) or a forceps (micro-Halstead or mosquito forceps), pick up the vein and pull it outside the skin.
- Ensure that you have picked up only the vein and nothing else.
- Apply two arterial clips to the vein, cut the vein between the forceps.
- Pull gently at each end until as much vein as possible has been pulled out, and avulse the vein.
- A "two forceps" technique is useful in pulling the vein. Apply one forceps and pull as much as possible and, while still pulling, apply a second forceps on the vein next to the skin. By repeating this, long segments of veins may be pulled out (see Figure 6.8, overleaf).
- Another technique is to apply an arterial clip and, by twisting the clip, the vein can be wrapped around the clip as it is being pulled out.
- There is no need to close these skin incisions. A small sticky plaster is adequate as a dressing. However, if required, Steristrips may be applied to approximate the edges of the wound.

6.10 Post-operative Care

At the end of the operation the leg is bandaged using crepe bandage. Usually three crepe bandages are needed: one 4-inch crepe around the foot and ankle and two 6-inch crepes around the leg and thigh, to the level of the highest phlebectomy or above the knee, whichever is higher. Ensure that the bandage is not too tight by checking capillary return at the toes, which should be left exposed. Keep the patient for a minimum

66 Manual of Ambulatory General Surgery

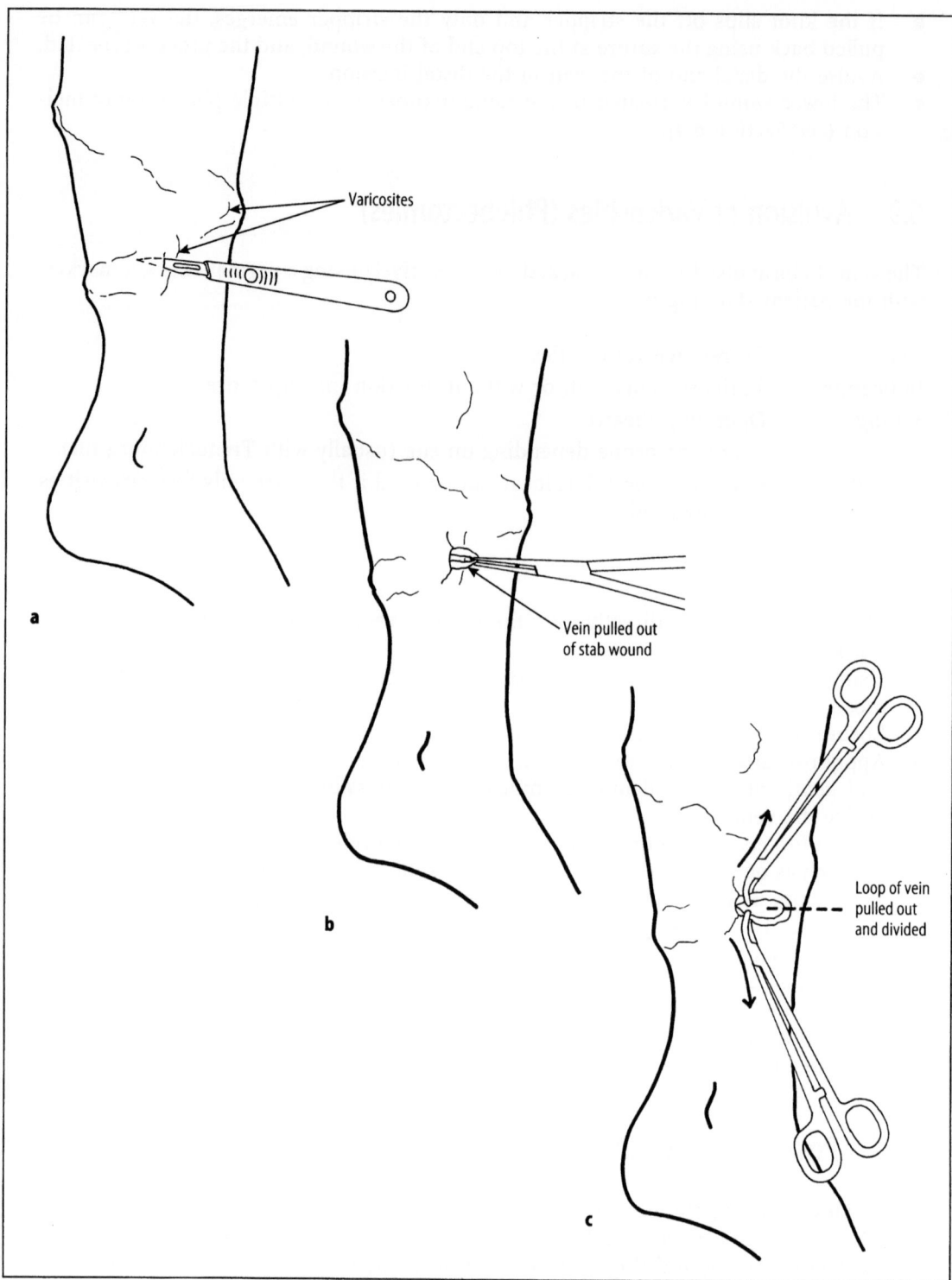

Figure 6.8 (This page and opposite).   Phlebectomies

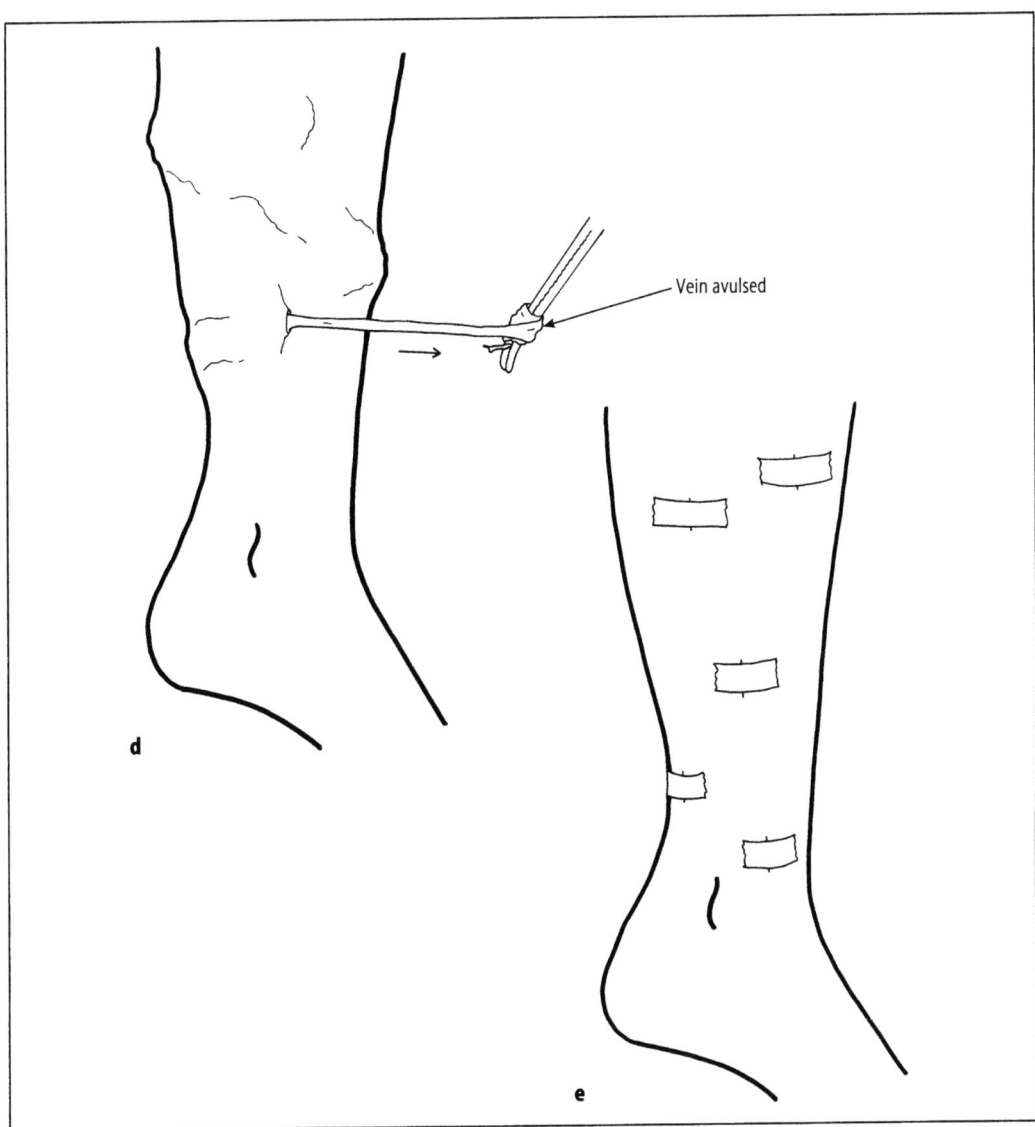

period of 3 hours post-operatively. Check the groin or popliteal incision (if there is one) for swelling or haematoma before discharging the patient.

We remove the crepe bandages and apply an above-knee compression stocking before discharging the patient. The patient is instructed to wear the compression stockings day and night for two weeks, and then only during the daytime for the next 4 weeks (ensure there is no arterial disease before compression stockings are used).

The patient is encouraged to walk as much as possible post-operatively. A review of the patient is done in the outpatient department 6 weeks after the operation. If any residual varicosities are found, they can be treated by sclerotherapy.

7 Hernia Repair

7.1 Introduction

This chapter describes the repair of uncomplicated primary inguinal, femoral and para-umbilical herniae in adults. Recurrent herniae, laparoscopic repairs and other more complicated hernia repairs are not discussed as we feel that it would be inappropriate for an SHO or GP to undertake these procedures. Only one safe and effective method of repair is described for each hernia. More comprehensive texts will need to be consulted for descriptions of other repairs.

7.2 Inguinal Hernia

Inguinal herniae may be direct or indirect. Sometimes both exist at the same time. More rarely a sliding hernia will be found. The following procedure is effective in all these situations. The hernia site must be clearly marked pre-operatively to avoid operating on the wrong side. It is probably inappropriate to operate on a bilateral hernia in a day-case setting.

Objective   To repair a primary (non-recurrent) inguinal hernia.
Indications   Inguinal hernia.
Setting   Operating theatre.
Position   Supine.
Anaesthetic   Local with sedation or general anaesthetic.

If local anaesthesia is to be used we recommend using sedation with 3 to 5 mg of intravenous Midazolam at the same time. Monitoring of the pulse, ECG, BP and O_2 saturation during the procedure is essential. We recommend the use of 50 to 60 ml of 0.25 per cent Bupivicaine (Marcaine). The skin and subcutaneous tissues are infiltrated before the skin incision, and as each layer is reached it is infiltrated before it is dissected out or manipulated.

Use prophylactic antibiotics (one dose immediately pre-operatively of a broad-spectrum antibiotic) as foreign material is going to be used for repair of the hernia.

Procedure
The operation can be broken down into a number of steps.

Exposure of the Cord

- Prepare the skin with an antiseptic solution and drape to expose the inguinal area.
- Feel for the anterior superior iliac spine and the pubic tubercle. A line drawn between these marks the position of the inguinal ligament.
- Make a skin crease incision about 7 cm long about 2 cm cranial to where you have determined the inguinal ligament to be.
- Cut through the skin, subcutaneous fat, Scarpa's fascia, and deep fat until you see the aponeurosis of the external oblique muscle. On route you will need to diathermy vessels to ensure haemostasis. (Sometimes Scarpa's fascia is thick – especially in children – and it may be mistaken for the external oblique.)
- Once you have identified the aponeurosis of the external oblique (with the fibres running medially and caudally), take a swab and push the fat off it in all directions so that you can clearly see about 4 cm of it in the cauda-cranial direction. The fat also needs to be swept off medially up the pubic tubercle.
- Put in a self-retaining retractor (use a Travis) to keep the edges of the wound apart.
- Identify the external ring. Inserting your index finger into it from the medial aspect best does this. If you are in the correct place, your finger should be able to travel 0.5 to 1 cm into the canal, making the anterior border of the external ring easier to identify.
- Make a small incision in the external oblique in the middle of the field of about 0.5 cm length and 2 cm cranial and parallel to the inguinal ligament.
- Attach an arterial clip to each side of the incision.
- Slide a pair of dissecting scissors (use McIndoe's) with the blades closed and the curvature facing upwards, and slide it just beneath the external oblique, progressing along the lines of the fibres medially towards the external ring. This manoeuvre separates the contents of the inguinal canal from the external oblique.
- Pull the scissors out. Now cut the external oblique from the small incision already made medially until the anterior border of the external ring has been cut.
- Repeat the above two steps, but this time go laterally up to the lateral extent of your skin incision.
- Lift up the caudal leaf of the external oblique using the attached arterial clip and use a swab to "clean" the internal surface off any tissue stuck to it. You should do this until you can see the inguinal ligament (the lower reflected edge of the external oblique aponeurosis) clearly from the pubic tubercle until the lateral edge of the incision.
- Repeat the above step for the cranial leaf of the external oblique until the conjoint tendon is revealed.
- Place the self-retaining retractor inside the inguinal canal, spreading the two leaves of the external oblique aponeurosis.
- The contents of the cord should be clearly visible.
- At this point the ilioinguinal nerve should be visible anterior to the cord. Dissect this nerve out carefully and protect it from damage during the operation. Moving it outside the operating field using the self-retaining retractor (separating the external oblique aponeurosis) may do this.
- Next, the spermatic cord must be separated from the floor of the inguinal canal. Do this with blunt dissection by
    - getting your index finger under the cord at the medial aspect as near to the pubic tubercle as possible; it may be necessary to lift the cord with one hand

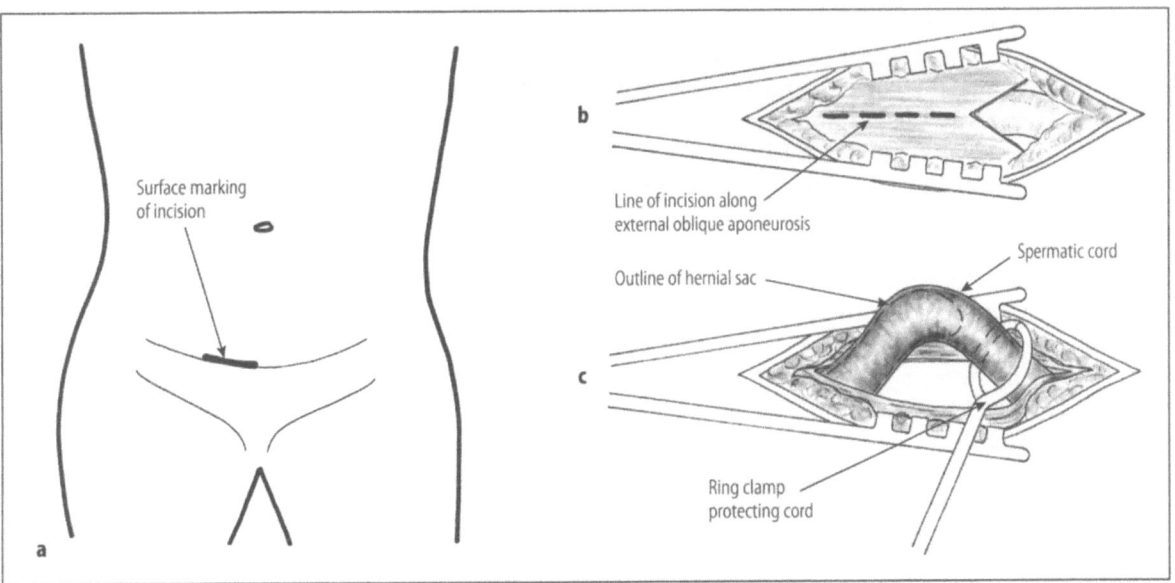

Figure 7.1. Incision and exposure of the cord

- (usually left) while trying to dissect with the index finger of the other hand (usually right)
  - hook the partially dissected cord using the index finger (right hand) and pull it away from the pubic tubercule and try to dissect the opposite side of the cord using the index finger of the other hand
  - keep doing this until both fingers meet behind the cord and the cord is separated from the floor of the inguinal canal
  - if you are using local anaesthesia you need to be gentle, as pulling on the cord tends to be painful.
- Apply a tissue clamp around the cord – use a hernia ring clamp or a Lane's tissue forceps. Ensure that the cord is not crushed by this manoeuvre. A catheter made into a loop using an arterial clip is an alternative to using a clamp.
- Lift the cord away from the body using the ring forceps and dissect the cord away from the rest of the floor of the inguinal canal by a mixture of sharp and blunt dissection in a lateral direction until the internal ring is reached. The cord should now be free from the floor of the inguinal canal from the internal ring to beyond the pubic tubercle.

Dissection of the Sac

- If the hernia is direct then you will see it in the floor of the inguinal canal behind the dissected-out cord. If the hernia sac is large and you feel that it will interfere with placement and suturing of the mesh (see below) then put in two or three interrupted sutures, plicating the floor of the inguinal canal (fascia tranversalis). Take very superficial bites from the caudal and cranial aspects of the fascia tranversalis using 3/0 Prolene or nylon. Even if the hernia is direct, it is advisable to examine in the cord for an indirect sac, as the two types of hernia may co-exist.

- The next step is to look for and dissect out an indirect sac (lying within the cord).
- To do this, first make an incision in the external cremasteric fascia (this is the fascia covering the cord) using scissors along the long axis of the cord.
- Cover your left index finger with a swab and place it under the cord and lift the cord away from the body, putting it on the stretch. Using your right hand with a swab pinched between your thumb and index finger, spread the contents of the cord (about 2 cm away from the internal ring) over the swab-covered index finger of the left hand. The aim is to identify the edge of an indirect sac.
- If you do not find the edge of the sac, repeat the process closer to the internal ring. If you have already found a direct hernia and there is still no sac at the internal ring (identified by the inferior epigastric vessels on the medial border of the ring) then there is no indirect hernia. In this case then skip the following steps and proceed to fixation of the mesh.
- If you have identified the edge of a sac, apply an arterial clip to it. Apply another arterial clip to the tissue stuck to the sac – ensure that you do not apply the clip on a vessel or the vas deferens.
- Take the arterial clip attached to the edge of the sac in your left hand and give the other arterial clip to an assistant. By pulling the two arterial clips apart, the plane of dissection between the sac and the rest of the tissue will be displayed. Use scissors to dissect away all the cord structures from the sac. The two arterial clips will need to be repositioned as you progress with the dissection. Do this until the sac is free of any tissue attached to it.
- Be especially careful not to damage the vas (which will be located posterior to the sac) and the surrounding blood vessels.
- If the sac is large and extending towards the scrotum, do not dissect it distally. You only need to dissect from the point of identification proximally to the internal ring.
- Continue dissecting the sac proximally until the internal ring. You will know you are there once you see the inferior epigastric vessels on the medial border of the internal ring or once you see the preperitoneal fat. Once you have dissected the sac up to the internal ring and it is free of any tissue attached to it, you have finished the dissection. Sometimes there is a fatty mass within the cord, often called "lipoma of the cord". If this is bulky, excise it and ensure haemostasis (its base may need transfixion). If it is small leave it alone.
- If the hernia sac is large and extends down the cord, transect the sac at a convenient location and apply two clips to the cut end (the distal part of the sac is to be left in situ). If the sac is small then it should be excised completely, apply two arterial clips to the apex of the sac about 0.5 cm apart and cut into the sac using scissors.
- Apply the clips to the edges of the cut sac and apply a third clip to the cut edge. Pull the three clips apart so that you can see the inside of the sac.
- If the sac has contents, try to reduce them back into the peritoneal cavity using a pair of wide jawed non-toothed forceps. Occasionally there are some adhesions between the contents and the sac. These need to be dissected out before the contents can be reduced. This is especially the case in a long-standing hernia. Be careful that you are not dealing with a sliding hernia (one where an extra-peritoneal organ, for example the large bowel, makes up part of the sac).
- If the hernia is not sliding and the contents of the sac have been reduced into the peritoneal cavity, then take the clips attached to the edges of the sac in one hand and start rotating them through several turns to "wring" the sac (see Figure 7.2b).

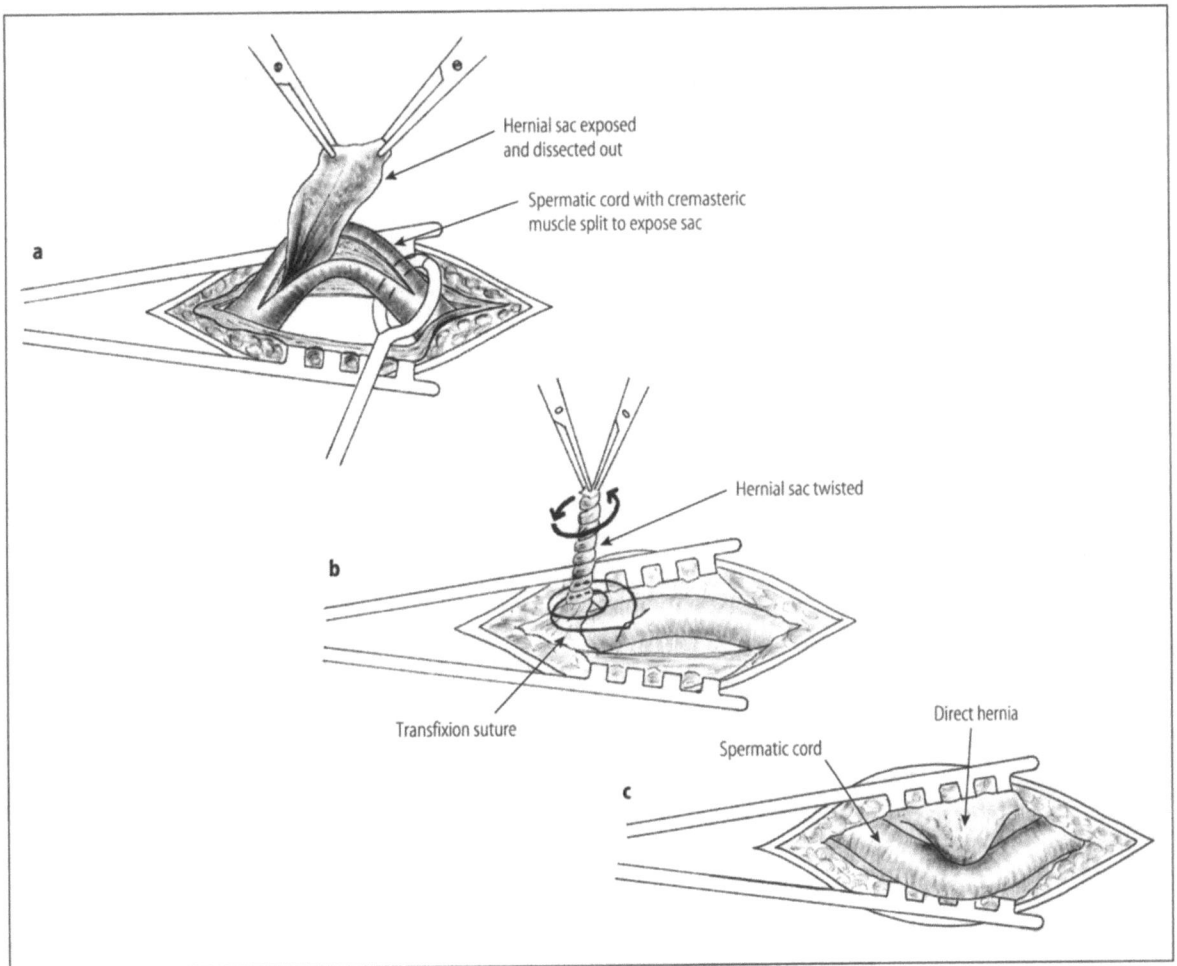

Figure 7.2. Dissection of the sac

This is to stop the contents re-entering the sac before transfixion of the base of the sac.
- Pull the clips up to put the sac on tension and transfix the cord at the base using 0 Vicryl on a round-bodied needle. (Transfixion means that the needle goes through the centre of the sac and the suture is tied on one side of the cord with a single throw and then the two ends of the suture are brought around the other side of the cord and tied securely. The purpose of transfixion, as opposed to simple tying, is to form a more secure knot.)
- Cut the excess sac, leave about 1 cm of sac beyond the tie, and cut the excess suture material. The base of the sac should disappear into the internal ring. Some surgeons prefer to attach the base of the sac to the underside of the conjoint tendon in the belief that this will reduce the chances of an indirect recurrence. To do this, do not cut both ends of the transfixtion suture – cut only the distal end, leaving the end with the needle attached intact. Insert the tip of the needle into the internal ring at the cranial end and bring it out through

the conjoint tendon. With the needle, take a bite of the conjoint tendon near where the suture emerged and tie the suture to itself and cut away the excess.
  ○ If the patient is female, it is possible to transfix and excise the "cord" as there are no structures of importance in it.
- If the hernia is a sliding hernia, cut the sac at a distance of about 1 cm from the sliding component. Place a purse string suture using 2/0 Vicryl along the cut edge of the sac. Pull on the two ends of the suture, closing the sac and tie the ends of the suture together. Now reduce the hernia through the internal ring.

Securing the Mesh

- The next step is shaping the mesh and securing it into position in the posterior wall of the inguinal canal.
- Take a piece of polypropelene mesh about 15 × 10 cm in size and cut it to make it the shape shown in Figure 7.3.
- Estimate the distance between the internal ring and the pubic tubercle add 1 cm to that estimate and create a slit and hole in the mesh through which the cord will pass as shown in Figure 7.3.
- Lay the mesh into the floor of the inguinal canal and place the cord through the slit into the hole in the mesh created for it.
- Get your assistant to expose the medial part of the mesh overlying the pubic tubercle with the help of one or two Langenbeck retractors.

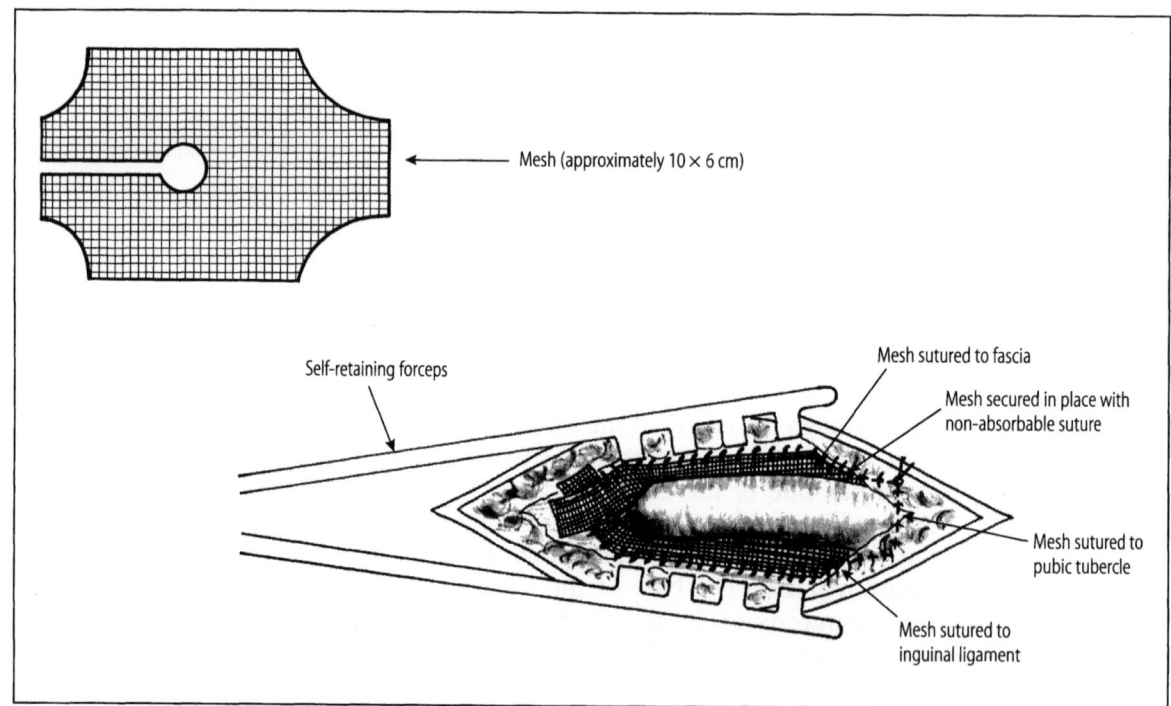

Figure 7.3. Shaping and securing the mesh

- Suture the mesh to the periosteum of the pubic tubercle by passing the needle through the mesh, through the tubercle then out through the mesh. Use 2/0 Prolene or nylon and tie the suture securely using at least seven throws. Leave the distal end of the suture about 10 cm long and apply an arterial clip to its end.
- Ask your assistant to retract the cord cranially, exposing the lower leaf of the mesh and the inguinal ligament. Suture the lower edge of the mesh to the inguinal ligament using a continuous suture. Take bites every half-centimetre until you are 1 cm lateral to the internal ring.
- Fold the cranial and lateral leaf of the mesh around the cord to overlap the caudal leaf and suture it to the inguinal ligament, and lock the suture by passing it through its own loop.
- Now suture the cranial leaf of the mesh to the conjoint tendon with a continuous suture from lateral to medial until you reach the pubic tubercle.
- Tie the proximal end of the suture to its distal end (previously attached to the arterial clip) using seven throws. Cut the excess suture material.
- The mesh should be lying in the floor of the canal under no tension and should be tenting in the middle slightly.
- Check that the hole in the mesh for the cord is snug. If it is not, then place a suture to tighten it. If, on the other hand, it is too tight and appears to be strangulating the cord, slit it medially.

Closure

- Ensure haemostasis using diathermy.
- Remove the self-retaining retractor from the inguinal canal and reposition it subcutaneously. This will expose the previously cut edges of the external oblique aponeurosis.
- Suture the external oblique aponeurosis from lateral to medial using a continuous 2/0 Vicryl suture. Make sure you do not narrow the external ring.
- Remove the self-retaining retractor.
- Apply three to four sutures to approximate Scarpa's fascia using 2/0 Vicryl on a round-bodied needle.
- Close the skin with a subcuticular suture (use a non-absorbable monofilament suture such as nylon or Prolene or an absorbable suture such as PDS or Vicryl).
- Apply an occlusive dressing.

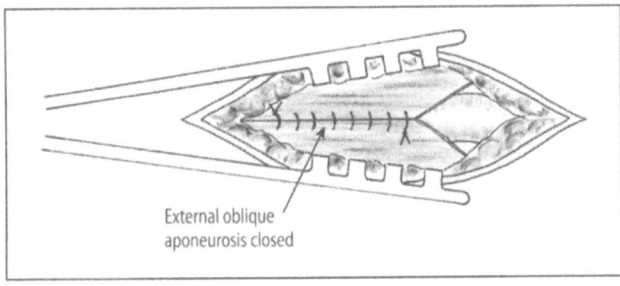

Figure 7.4. Closing the external oblique over the cord

- In the male, pull the testis down to the bottom of the scrotum. (The testis may have been pulled up to the top of the scrotum as a result of traction on the cord during the operation.)
- Sutures should be removed in 7 days if non-absorbable sutures have been used.

7.3 Femoral Hernia

Femoral herniae are usually irreducible and are not uncommon, especially in females. The description below relates to an elective repair of a femoral hernia.

Objective To repair a primary (non-recurrent) femoral hernia electively (non-emergency).
Indications Femoral hernia.
Setting Operating theatre.
Position Supine, with legs spread apart.
Anaesthetic Local anaesthetic with sedation or general anaesthetic.

If local anaesthesia is to be used we recommend using sedation with 3 to 5 mg of intravenous Midazolam at the same time. Monitoring of the pulse, ECG, BP and O_2 saturation during the procedure is essential. We recommend the use of 50 to 60 ml of 0.25 per cent Bupivicaine (Marcaine). The skin and subcutaneous tissues are infiltrated before the skin incision, and as each layer is reached it is infiltrated before it is dissected out or manipulated.

Procedure

- Prepare and drape the area to expose the femoral area.
- Palpate the hernia and make a transverse skin incision of about 5 cm over it.
- Carefully cut down through the subcutaneous fat until the hernial sac is reached. This is easy to recognise as it separates off the surrounding fat easily.
- Grasp the hernia sac with a pair of broad non-toothed forceps or with a tissue grasping forceps (for example Allis forceps) and dissect the sac off the tissue surrounding it. Use a combination of sharp dissection with scissors and blunt dissection using a Layhe swab to clear the fat off the sac.
- Continue doing this cranially until the neck of the sac is reached. The neck of the sac is formed by the femoral vein laterally, the lacunar ligament medially, the inguinal ligament anteriorly and the pubic ramus and pectineal ligament posteriorly.
- Apply two arterial clips to the apex of the sac and open the sac to inspect the contents. Often you will only find fat in the sac.
- Push any contents back into the peritoneal cavity. If the contents are adherent to the sac you may need to release these adhesions.
- If it is difficult to reduce the contents, the neck of the sac may need to be enlarged. Do this by inserting a pair of scissors (use McIndoe's) with the blades closed along the medial edge of the sac into the neck of the hernial defect (the scissors should

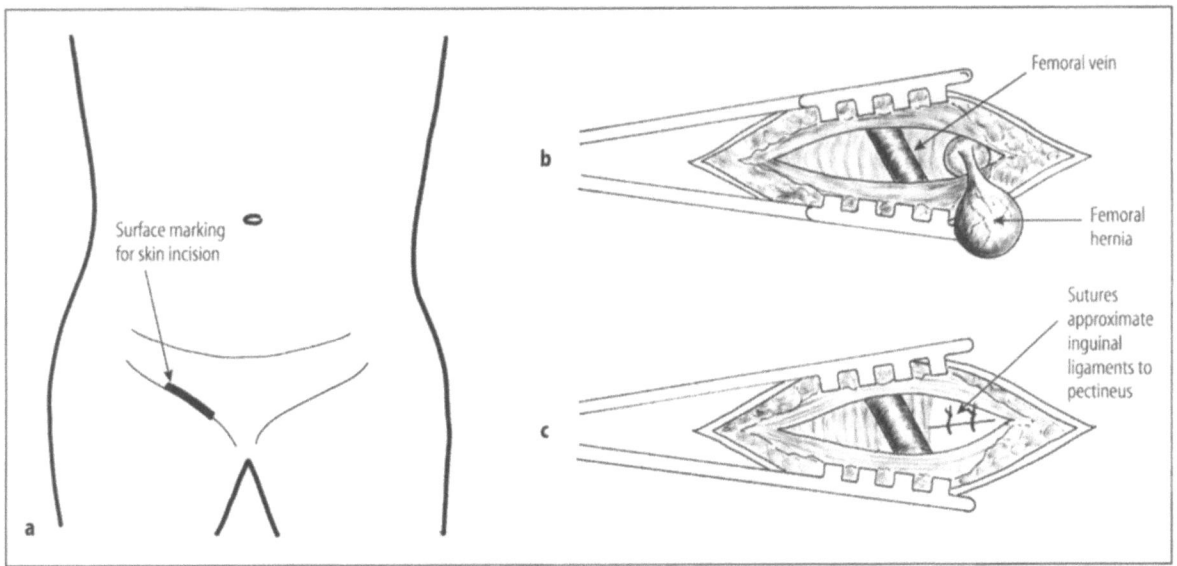

Figure 7.5. Femoral hernia repair

be outside and not inside the sac). Gently open the blades to dilate the neck. Try reducing the contents again. If you fail you may need to dilate further.
- Once you have reduced the contents, take the two arterial clips on the apex of the sac and rotate them a number of times, thus wringing the sac.
- Apply a transfixion stitch at the neck of the sac and excise the redundant sac.
- Place two or three interrupted sutures approximating the anterior and posterior edges of the hernial defect using 0 monofilament non-absorbable sutures (for example Prolene). Tie the sutures after all of them are in place. Be careful not to damage the femoral vein lateral to the defect.
- Ensure that there is no defect left.
- Close the fat with 2/0 Vicryl on a round-bodied needle.
- Close the skin with a subcuticular suture (use a non-absorbable monofilament suture such as nylon or Prolene or a monofilament absorbable suture such as PDS).
- Arrange for sutures to be removed in 7 days if non-absorbable sutures have been used.

7.4 Para-umbilical Hernia

Objective   To repair a primary (non-recurrent) para-umbilical hernia.
Indications   Para-umbilical hernia.
Setting   Operating theatre.
Position   Supine.
Anaesthetic   General.

Procedure

- Prepare and drape the area to expose the umbilical area.
- Palpate the hernia and decide if the defect is supra-umbilical or infra-umbilical (this can also be determined pre-operatively by careful examination).
- Make a transverse slightly curved infra-umbilical incision for an infra-umbilical hernia, or a transverse supra-umbilical incision for a supra-umbilical hernia.
- Carefully cut down through the subcutaneous fat until the hernial sac is reached. This is easy to recognise as it separates off the surrounding fat easily.
- Grasp the hernia sac with a pair of broad non-toothed forceps or with a tissue grasping forceps (for example Allis forceps) and dissect the sac off the tissue surrounding it. Use a combination of sharp dissection with scissors and blunt dissection using a Layhe swab to clear the fat off the sac.
- Continue doing this until the neck of the sac is reached. Usually the defect is quite small.
- Dissect the defect until the edges are clearly defined.
- If the sac is small and empty, reduce it through the defect. If it is large and appears to have contents, apply two arterial clips to the apex, open it, reduce the contents and transfix it at the base as described for a femoral hernia.
- If the sac is difficult to reduce, the defect may need to be widened. To do this, make a slit in it in the horizontal plane using scissors.
- To repair the defect, apply an Allis clamp to each side of the defect. Place a number of interrupted sutures (monofilament non-absorbable 0 sutures). Tie the sutures after all of them have been placed.
- For large defects (greater than 3 cm) the two edges of the defect may need to be made to overlap (Mayo repair). To do this, two rows of sutures are needed: one

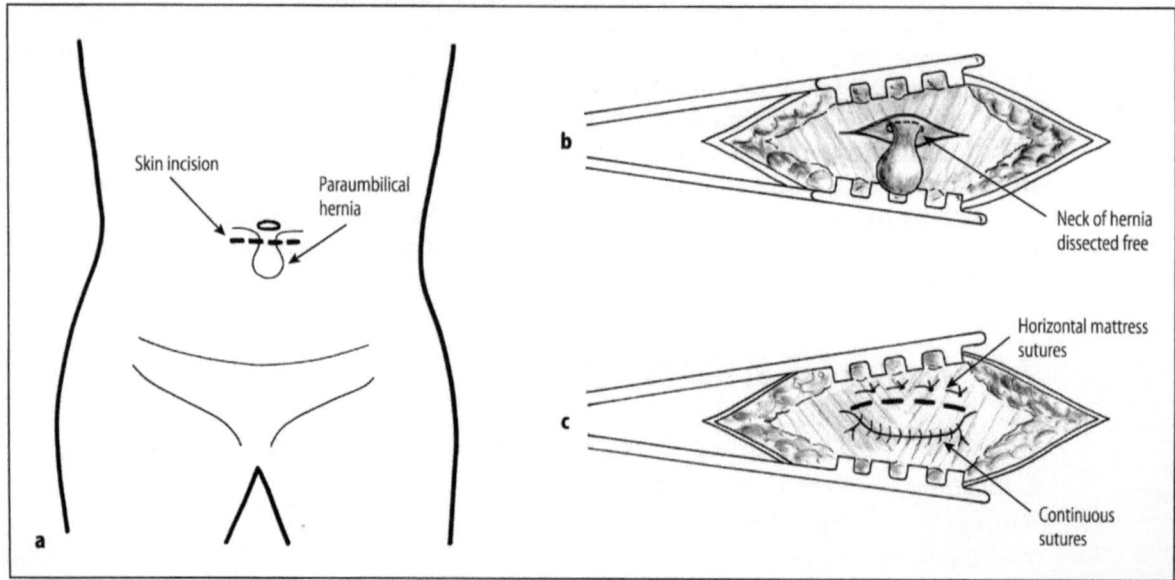

Figure 7.6. Para-umbilical hernia repair

row suturing one edge of the defect to the undersurface of the other edge, and another row suturing the top edge to the anterior aspect of the lower edge. Place all the sutures in each row before tying them (use monofilament non-absorbable 0 sutures).
- If during the dissection the whole of the umbilicus needs to be freed from the underlying tissue, it is advisable to tack the umbilicus to the fascia in order to reconstruct the umbilicus. Do this by passing a non-absorbable suture though the dermis of the umbilical skin deep to the umbilicus and suture it to the underlying fascia.
- Close the fat layer with interrupted 2/0 Vicryl if needed.
- Close the skin with a subcuticular suture (use a non-absorbable monofilament suture such as nylon or Prolene or a monofilament absorbable suture such as PDS).
- Arrange for sutures to be removed in 7 days if non-absorbable sutures have been used.

7.5 Other Herniae

Other abdominal-wall herniae such as epigastric herniae can be tackled in exactly the same way as a para-umbilical hernia. More complex herniae such as incisional or recurrent herniae should not be tackled by an SHO or GP except if supervised.

8 Anal Procedures

8.1 Introduction

Most anal procedures can be done on a day-case basis. For most of the procedures it is preferable, though not essential, to have the rectum empty. This can be achieved by the use of suppositories several hours before the procedure and an enema an hour prior to the procedure. Procedures that require specialist training such as colonoscopy or in-patient treatment, such as haemorrhoidectomy, have not been included.

8.2 Investigative Procedures

8.2.1 Proctoscopy

Objective To examine the anal canal and lower rectum.
Indication When pathology in the area is suspected.
Setting Outpatient clinic setting or in the operating theatre.
Preparation No preparation is needed.
Anaesthetic None needed.
Position For this procedure the patient may be in one of the following positions:
- the left lateral position (lying on the left side with the knees bent up to the chest and the feet forwards)
- the lithotomy position (lying on the back, with the hips flexed and the knees flexed and the feet supported in straps)
- the jack-knife position (patient prone and resting on knees and elbows with the hips and knees flexed).

Usually, if the patient is awake, the left lateral position is used, and if the patient is under anaesthetic, the lithotomy position is used.

The jack-knife position is only used by some surgeons for certain types of anal operations.

Procedure
- Check the instruments; in particular, that the light source is working. If any further procedure such as injection of haemorrhoids is to be undertaken, ensure that all the equipment is ready.

- Do a digital examination of the rectum (do not forget to use a lubricant such as K-Y Jelly).
- Insert the obturator in the proctoscope, lubricate the end, and gently insert the proctoscope into the rectum as far as it will go under direct vision.
- Remove the obturator and connect the light source.
- Examine the rectum and anal canal as the proctoscope is withdrawn.

8.2.2 Rigid Sigmoidoscopy

Objective To examine the rectum and recto-sigmoid junction, and sometimes it is possible to examine the lower sigmoid colon.
Indication When pathology in the area is suspected or needs to be excluded.
Setting Outpatient clinic setting or in the operating theatre.
Preparation No preparation is usually needed, but suppositories or a disposable enema can be used.
Anaesthetic None needed.
Position As for proctoscopy (see Section 8.2.1).

Procedure

- Check the instruments; in particular, that the light source is working, that the end-piece fits the sigmoidoscope, and that the insufflation works. Ensure that biopsy forceps are available. In some circumstances suction may be needed.
- Do a digital examination of the rectum (do not forget to use a lubricant such as K-Y Jelly).
- Insert the obturator in the sigmoidoscope, lubricate the end, and gently insert the sigmoidoscope into the rectum (aiming towards the umbilicus) under direct vision until resistance is felt (about 5 cm).
- Remove the obturator and connect the end-piece and switch on the light source.
- Look into the sigmoidoscope, and withdraw backwards 1 to 2 cm while insufflating.
- You should now be able to see a rectal fold. Direct the sigmoidoscope forwards and try to get round the fold. Further insufflation should reveal the next fold to go around.
- Go as high up as you can go without endangering the patient (only advance the sigmoidoscope forward if you can see where you are going) or causing too much discomfort.
- Examine the rectum as you slowly withdraw the instrument.
- Use the minimum of insufflation during the procedure to reduce the risk of perforation and patient discomfort.

Difficulties

- If you do not see the direction to head in, withdraw the sigmoidoscope a few centimetres and start again.
- If there are solid faeces, pass the sigmoidoscope alongside the faeces next to the bowel wall.
- If there are liquid faeces/enema fluid, use suction with a long rigid end-piece, or small pieces of cotton wool passed up the sigmoidoscope with the biopsy forceps.

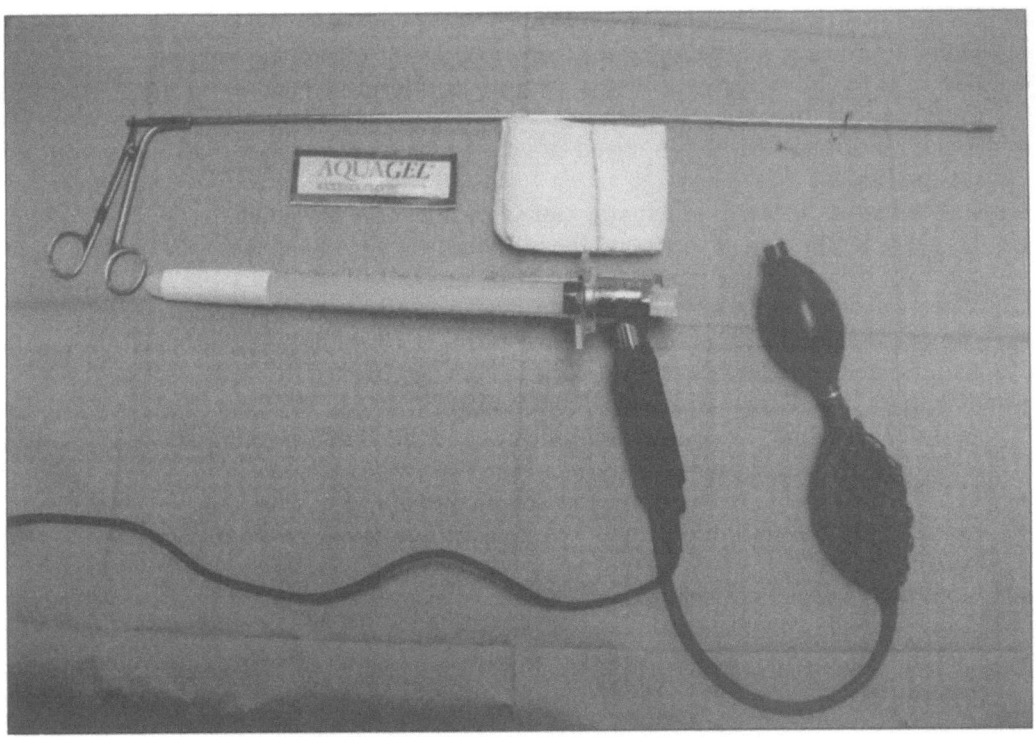

Figure 8.1. Equipment needed for rigid sigmoidoscopy

8.2.3 Flexible Sigmoidoscopy

Objective   To examine the rectum, sigmoid colon and descending colon.

Indication   When pathology in the area is suspected or needs to be excluded as well as when pathology has been diagnosed on barium enema and a biopsy or removal of a lesion such as a polyp is to be undertaken.

Setting   Outpatient clinic setting, endoscopy suite or in the operating theatre.

Preparation   A disposable enema one hour prior to examination – some surgeons do not recommend any preparation as solid faeces can be easily negotiated.

Anaesthetic   None needed. Pethidine IV (50 to 75 mg) may be given in cases of patient discomfort. An IV hypnotic such as Midazolam (2 to 5 mg) may also be used. If sedation is used we recommend the patient is monitored with a pulse oximeter during the procedure. Oxygen at 4 l/m should also be given through a nasal route or mask.

Position   As for proctoscopy (see Section 8.2.1).

Procedure

- Check the instruments, in particular that the light source, suction, air and water supply are working.

- Do a digital examination of the rectum.
- Lubricate the end of the sigmoidoscope and insert it into the rectum.
- Use insufflation to see where you are (try to minimise your use of insufflation to avoid patient discomfort).
- If you do not see the lumen ahead of you, draw the instrument back until you can see the lumen.
- Only advance forwards when you can see where you are going.
- To get a better idea of the way ahead, bend the tip of the instrument with your controls, then twist the scope itself in a clockwise then anticlockwise direction. This allows you to look in all directions to determine the way forwards.
- The recto-sigmoid junction will cause problems for the inexperienced, but with training and practice it becomes easier.
- If there is diverticular disease present, ensure that you are sure you are going up the lumen and not up a diverticulum (only advance the instrument when you can see where you are going).
- You should be able to get up to the splenic flexure.
- Examine the bowel lining on the way out, withdrawing the instrument slowly and looking carefully.
- Biopsy any suspicious lesions for histological examination and document where the biopsy is from (distance from anus).
- Examine the patient and ensure that there are no signs of peritonitis following the procedure.

Notes

- If the procedure is being done to assess colitis, take biopsies from all areas of the colon and put them in separate labelled pots.
- Do not do any biopsies if the patient is anticoagulated.
- If there is severe patient discomfort abandon the procedure.
- If you cannot see where you are going abandon the procedure.

8.3 Examination under Anaesthesia (EUA)

Objective   To examine the perianal area, anal canal and rectum.
Indication   When it has been impossible to do the examination in an outpatient clinic, or prior to an ano-rectal procedure.
Setting   Operating theatre.
Preparation   Suppositories or a disposable enema (for example phosphate enema) prior to the procedure.
Anaesthetic   General.
Position   Usually lithotomy, though left lateral or jack-knife may be used.

Procedure

- Spread the buttocks and do a careful external examination of the anus and perineum looking for:

- any sign of swelling and inflammation indicative of an abscess
  - any external opening on the skin, possibly with pus oozing out indicative of a fistula-in-ano; if you see this try and feel for a subcutaneous tract leading to the anus/rectum
  - skin tags
  - an anal fissure
  - an anal carcinoma
  - ulceration
  - thread worms.
- Apply some lubricant on your index finger and palpate the edges of the anal canal for signs of scarring subcutaneously, especially in the case of a fistula-in-ano, as you may be able to feel the tract subcutaneously.
- Do a digital examination of the anal canal and lower rectum feeling for mucosal or submucosal lesions.
- Do a proctoscopy as described in Section 8.2.1.
- Do a sigmoidoscopy as described in Sections 8.2.2–3.
- Note down all your findings.

8.4 Haemorrhoids

Objective To eliminate haemorrhoids.
Indications Symptomatic haemorrhoids. The indications for surgery are haemorrhoids that have not responded to conservative therapy or other modes of therapy (i.e. injections or banding), or third degree haemorrhoids (always prolapsed).
Setting Injections and banding are normally performed in an outpatient setting.
Preparation None needed.
Anaesthetic None needed.
Position Left lateral.

8.4.1 Injection of Haemorrhoids

Procedure

- Prepare the proctoscope and injection (use a maximum of 5 ml of phenol in almond oil for each haemorrhoid – about 3 ml should be the usual amount used).
- Insert the proctoscope as described in Section 8.2.1.
- Identify haemorrhoids by slowly retracting the proctoscope and watching them bulge inwards.
- Identify Hilton's white line.
- Identify the pedicle to the haemorrhoids above Hilton's white line.
- Inject up to 3 ml of phenol into the pedicle of the haemorrhoid submucosally above Hilton's white line. (Deeper injection anteriorly in the male may go into the prostate, causing prostatitis and haematuria.)
- The patient should only feel minimal discomfort; if the procedure is painful the injection is too low (distal).

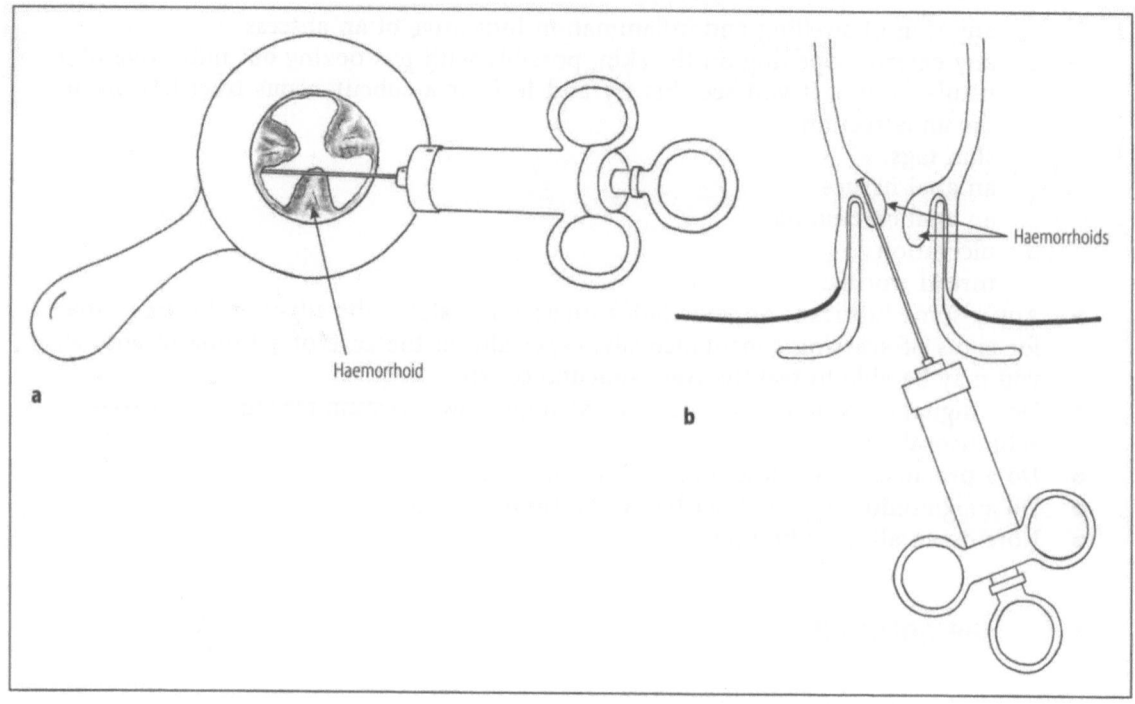

Figure 8.2. Injection of haemorrhoids

- Record which haemorrhoids were injected.
- Warn the patient that some bleeding may occur over the following few days as a result of the injection.
- Ask the patient to attend for further examination/repeat injection in 6 weeks' time.
- Up to three sessions of injections may be needed to treat the haemorrhoids.

8.4.2 Banding of Haemorrhoids

Procedure

- Prepare the proctoscope and load up three "banders"
- Insert the proctoscope as described in Section 8.2.1.
- Identify haemorrhoids by slowly retracting the proctoscope and watching them bulge inwards.
- Identify Hilton's white line.
- Identify the pedicle to the haemorrhoids above Hilton's white line.
- Put a grasping forceps through the centre of the bander and advance forceps into the proctoscope.
- Grasp the pedicle of the haemorrhoid with the forceps.
- Pull the pedicle gently while advancing the bander until it is around the pedicle.
- Fire the bander.

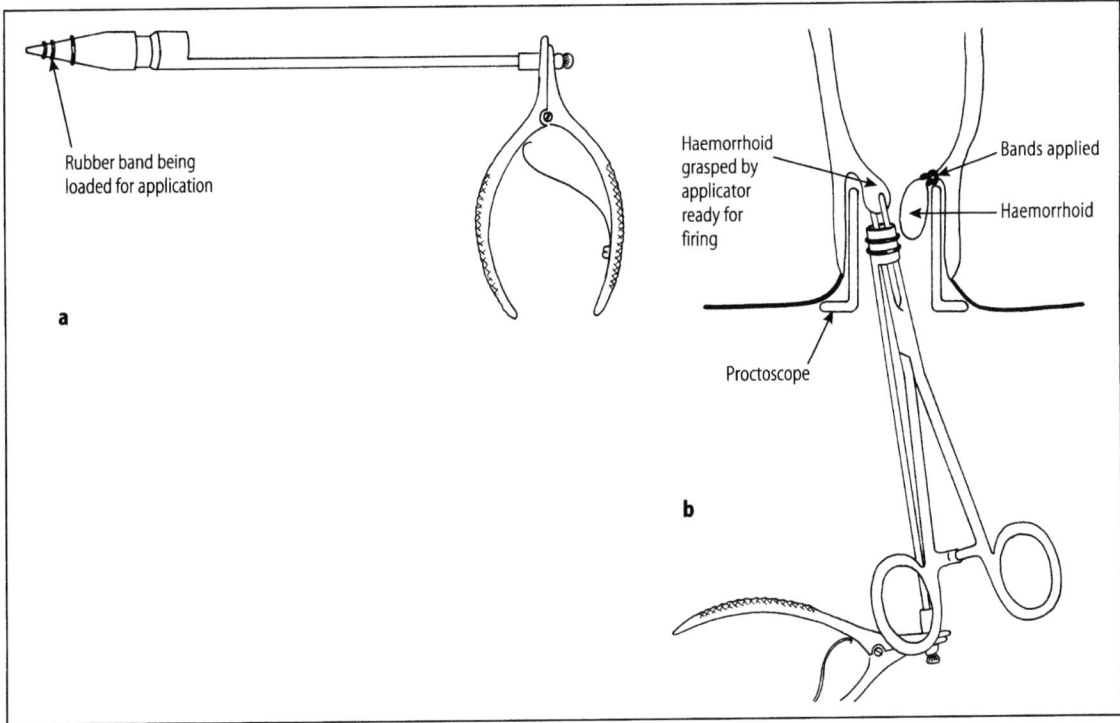

Figure 8.3. Banding of haemorrhoids

- Release the forceps and withdraw it out of the proctoscope along with the bander.
- Ensure visually that banding of the pedicle has occurred.
- Progress to band up to three haemorrhoids at one session.
- If the banding is painful, then you are doing it too low.
- If pain persists, remove the band and apply higher.
- Record which haemorrhoids have been banded.
- Warn the patient that some bleeding may occur about 10 days later (when the pedicle of the pile necroses and the band falls out).
- Ask the patient to attend for further examination/banding in 6 weeks' time.

8.5 Skin Tags

Objective   To excise symptomatic skin tags.
Indication   Itching, bleeding, discomfort due to skin tags.
Setting   Operating theatre.
Preparation   None needed.
Anaesthetic   General anaesthesia, although it is possible to perform this under local anaesthesia if the tags are small.
Position   Lithotomy.

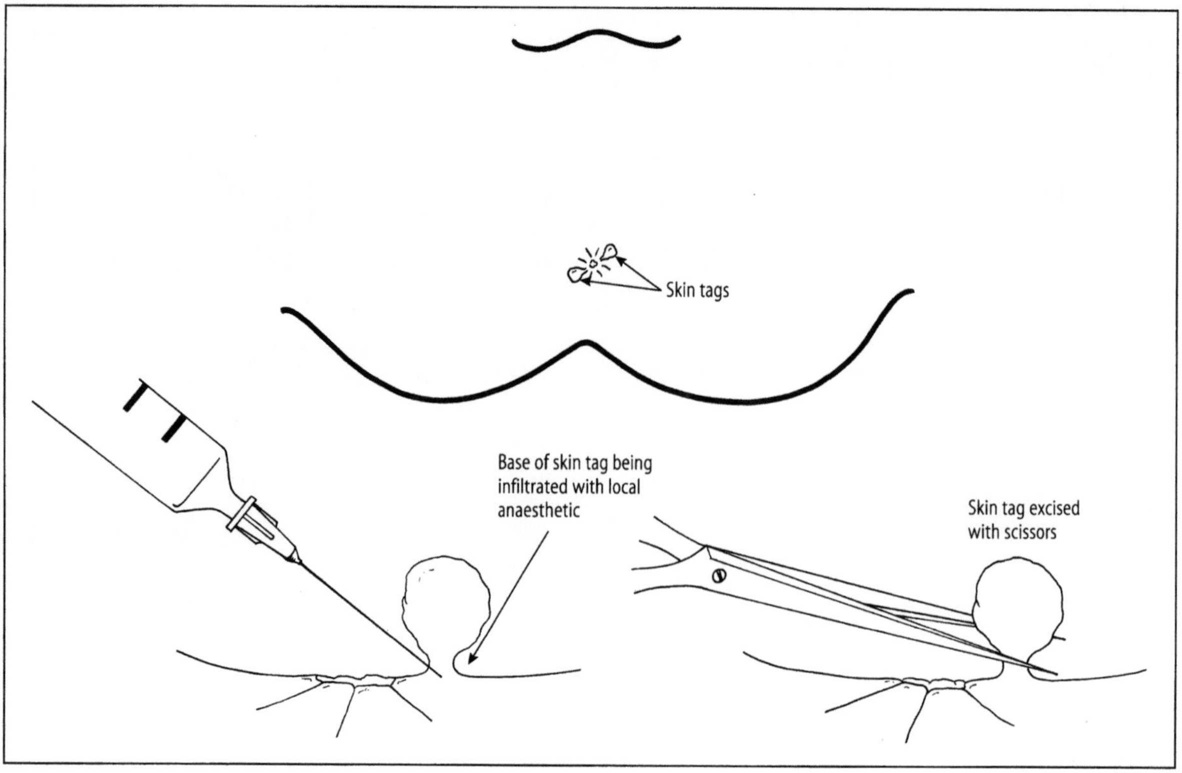

Figure 8.4. Excision of skin tags

Procedure

- Do an EUA as described in Section 8.3.
- Identify the tags to be excised.
- Infiltrate subcutaneously with 1 to 5 ml of 0.5 per cent Marcaine with 1:200,000 adrenaline (warn the anaesthetist before you do this).
- Grasp the tag with a pair of toothed forceps.
- Make an elliptical cut around the "tag" at the anal margin, using scissors.
- Dissect the tag off the subcutaneous tissue; the local infiltration should have lifted the tag off for you.
- Secure haemostasis with diathermy if needed.
- Cover each site with a piece of tulle impregnated with paraffin. (We do not normally close the wound, but this can be done with an absorbable suture such as 2/0 Vicryl if required.)
- Prescribe laxatives post-operatively (Fybogel or Lactulose).

8.6 Anal Fissure

Objective   To cure an anal fissure by preventing the internal anal sphincter from functioning, and thus relieving anal spasm.

Indication	Anal fissure.
Setting	Operating theatre.
Preparation	None needed.
Anaesthetic	General anaesthesia, though lateral (internal) sphincterotomy can be performed under local anaesthesia.
Position	Usually lithotomy.

8.6.1 Anal Stretch

Procedure

- Do an EUA as described in Section 8.3.
- Determine any other pathology (such as fistula-in-ano, haemorrhoids etc.) and treat appropriately.
- Apply a generous quantity of lubricating jelly (such as K-Y Jelly) onto the index finger of the left hand.
- Insert the left index finger into the anal canal.
- Apply some lubricating jelly onto the index finger of the right hand.
- Insert the right index finger into the anal canal.
- Stretch the anal canal to allow insertion of another finger.
- Withdraw the left index finger and now insert both the index and middle fingers of the left hand into the anal canal.
- Stretch the anal canal to allow insertion of another finger.
- Withdraw the right index finger and now insert both the index and middle fingers of the right hand into the anal canal.
- You should now have four fingers in the anal canal.

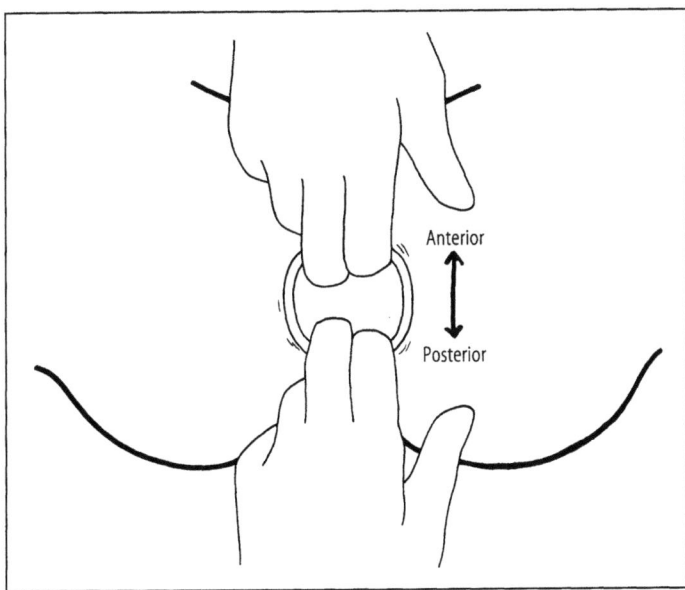

Figure 8.5. Anal stretch

- Do a further gentle stretch so that the total diameter of the anal canal is 5 to 6 cm.
- Prescribe laxatives post-operatively (Fybogel or Lactulose).

Notes

- The "classical" anal stretch is an eight-finger stretch. However, this has an unacceptably high complication rate of faecal incontinence, and so we recommend a four-finger stretch if a stretch is to be done at all.
- Lateral (internal) sphincterotomy is a much better procedure for this condition.
- If there is any possibility of the patient suffering from Crohn's disease (multiple fissures, painless fissures, previous abscesses, etc.), do not do this procedure as faecal incontinence may occur. Refer this patient to a specialist.

8.6.2 Lateral (Internal) Sphincterotomy

Procedure

- Do an EUA as described in Section 8.3.
- Determine any other pathology (such as fistula-in-ano, haemorrhoids etc.) and treat appropriately.
- Insert a Park's retractor into the anal canal after lubricating it (do not use the third blade of the retractor).
- Open the retractor in the anal canal with one blade at the top of the anal canal (anteriorly) and the opposite blade at the bottom (posteriorly).
- This will allow access to the lateral aspect of the anal canal.
- Palpate with your right index finger from within the anal canal on the left side of the patient outwards.
- About 0.5 cm from the anal verge a groove will be encountered. This is the groove between the internal and external anal sphincter. Inject local anaesthetic with adrenaline to minimise bleeding (use 5 ml of 0.5 per cent Marcaine with 1:200,000 Epinephrine).
- Make a vertical incision of about 7 mm using a no. 15 blade where the groove was palpated.
- Insert curved scissors (with the blades closed and the tip pointing medially) between the internal and external sphincter to a depth of about 2 cm.
- Withdraw the scissors and re-insert it through the same incision, but now between the internal sphincter and the mucosa of the anal canal (keep the tip facing laterally) to a depth of about 2 cm.*
- Withdraw the scissors and insert an arterial clip into the previously created space between the internal and external sphincters.

---

* At this point some surgeons recommend putting in the blades of the scissors into the spaces created on either side of the internal sphincter and cutting it. Other surgeons recommend putting in a scalpel mounted with a no. 15 blade into the wound, passing it up the space created between the internal and external sphincters (keeping the blade vertical) then turning the blade through 90 degrees medially (towards the anus) and cutting the internal sphincter (care must be taken not to cut all the way through into the anus).

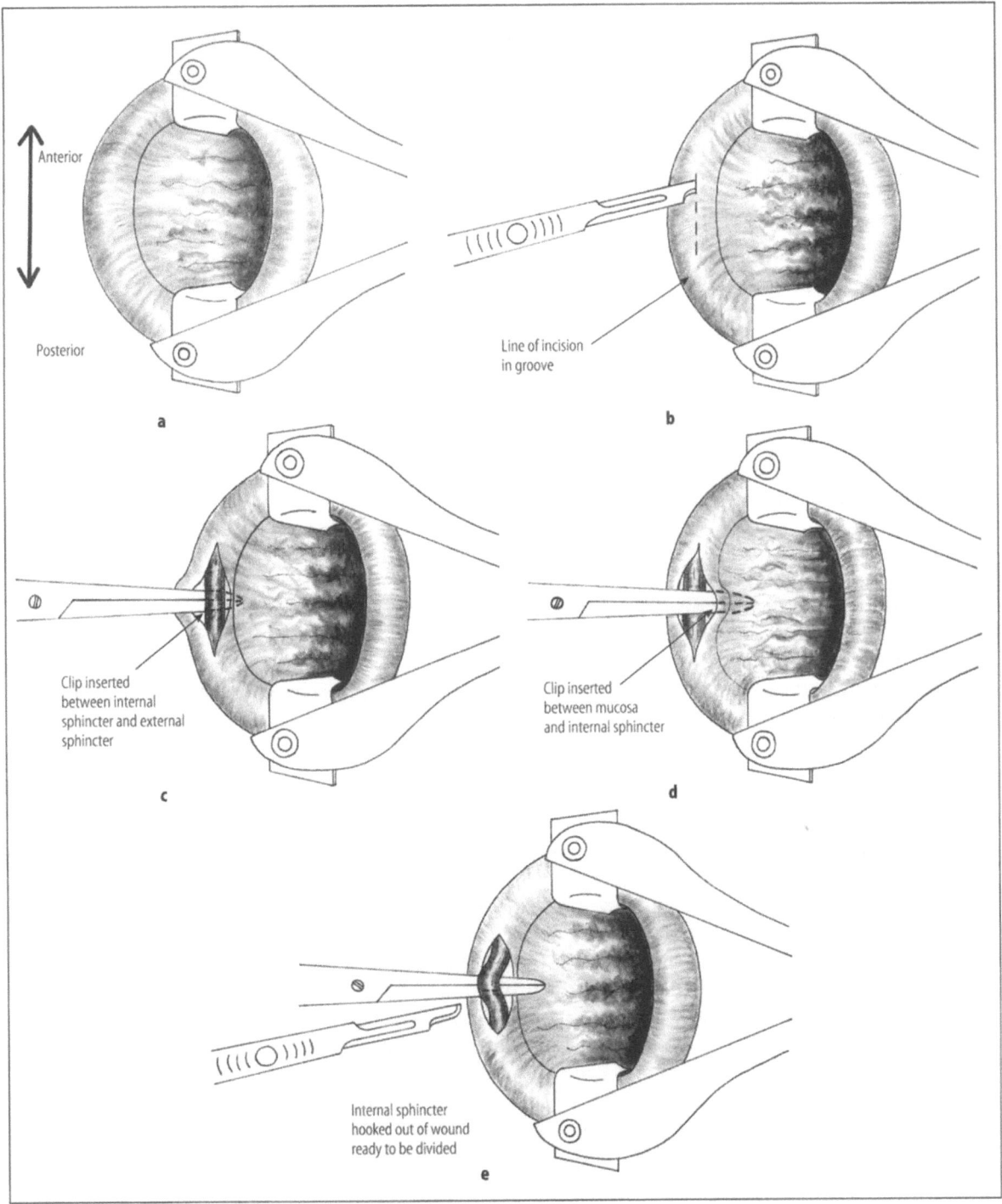

Figure 8.6. Lateral sphincterotomy

- Turn the tip medially and hook the internal sphincter so that the tip of the forceps re-emerges out of the incision, pulling out with it the internal sphincter.
- Cut the internal sphincter with scissors or scalpel blade.
- Ensure that there are no further fibres of the internal sphincter left by trying to hook them out.
- Apply tulle gauze impregnated with paraffin.
- Prescribe laxatives post-operatively (Fybogel or Lactulose).

8.7 Fistula-in-Ano

Objective   To cure a fistula-in-ano by laying open the tract and allowing it to heal by granulation.
Indication   Fistula-in-ano.
Setting   Operating theatre.
Preparation   None needed.
Anaesthetic   General.
Position   Lithotomy.

Procedure: Fistulotomy – Laying Open of Fistula-in-Ano

- Do an EUA as described in Section 8.3.
- During the proctoscopy try and determine the internal opening of the fistula (you may see some pus coming out of it).
- Determine any other pathology (such as an anal fissure, haemorrhoids etc.) and treat appropriately.
- Determine the external opening of the fistula.
- Lubricate the index finger of your right hand and palpate between the external opening and the anal canal to try and feel the "tract" of the fistula.
- Apply Goodsall's law to determine where the internal opening is likely to be. This law states that if an imaginary line is drawn horizontally though the middle of the anus (1) a fistula with an external opening below (posterior to) the line, the internal opening will lie in the mid-line posteriorly (tract curving posteriorly), (2) whereas, a fistula with an external opening above this line the internal opening will lie at the same level as the external opening (straight tract).
- Insert a blunt probe (lacrimal duct probe may be used) into the external opening of the fistula and gently guide it through the tract until it emerges out of the internal opening. Ensure that you do not force the probe through the mucosa thus creating a new tract.
- Determine if this is a low or high fistula. A low fistulous tract will be subcutaneous or, if not, will only include a small portion of the external sphincter. If you are in any doubt, treat it as a high fistula.

Low Fistula

- At this stage you should have the probe going through the external opening and coming out of the internal opening.

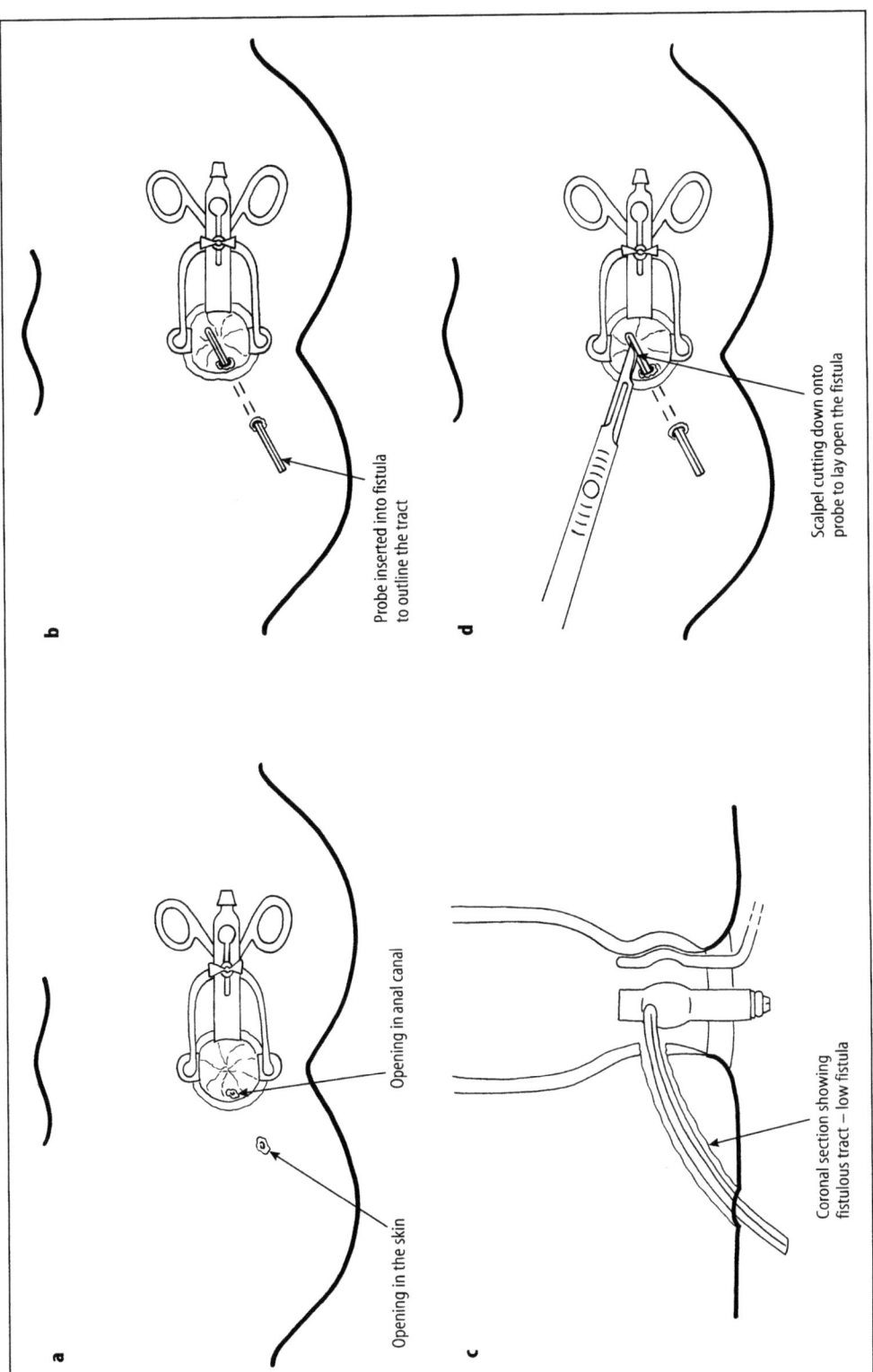

Figure 8.7. Laying open of fistula-in-ano (low fistula)

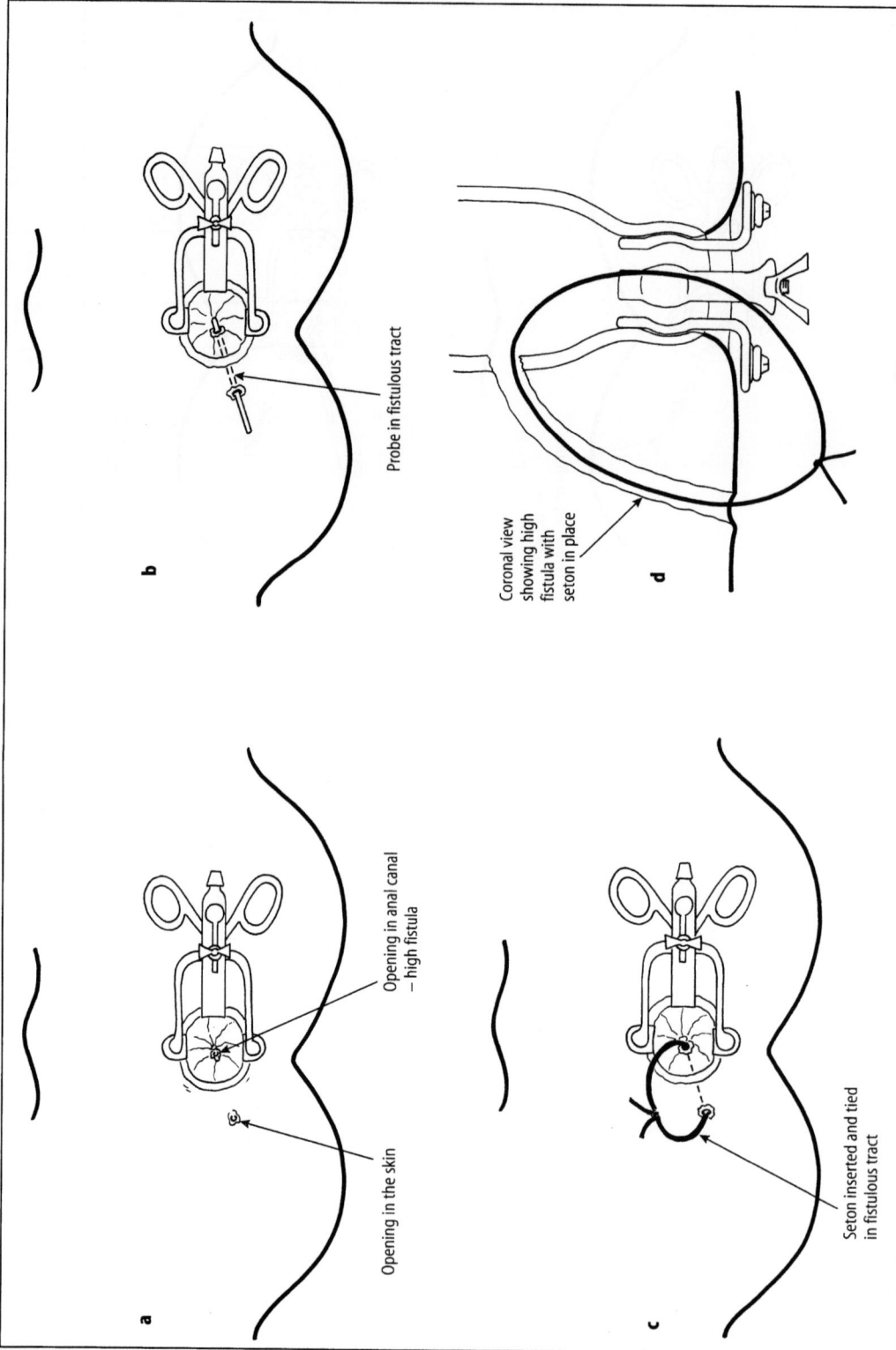

Figure 8.8. Seton insertion

- If it is a grooved probe, turn the probe so that the groove is facing you.
- Inject local anaesthetic with adrenaline into the tissue around the tract to minimise bleeding (use 5 ml of 0.5 per cent Bupivicaine with 1:200,000 adrenaline).
- Using a no. 15 blade, cut down onto the probe from the external to the internal opening until the probe is released.
- Remove a bit of the tract and send it for histology.
- Curette the tract of the fistula.
- Apply tulle gauze impregnated with paraffin.
- Prescribe laxatives post-operatively (Fybogel or Lactulose).

High Fistula

- At this stage you should have the probe going through the external opening and coming out of the internal opening.
- If you feel this is a high fistula do not lay it open as you may cause faecal incontinence.
- Tie a heavy tie (such as no. 1 silk) to the end of the probe and pull the probe out pulling the suture through the tract. The suture should now be going through the tract of the fistula with one end of it coming out of the internal opening and the other end out of the external opening. Tie the suture tightly and securely and cut the ends, leaving them long. This procedure is called a Seton procedure.
- Refer the patient on for specialist treatment.

8.8 Anal Warts

Objective	To eliminate anal warts.
Indication	Anal warts.
Setting	Operating theatre.
Preparation	None needed.
Anaesthetic	Local if there are only a few, otherwise general.
Position	Lithotomy.

Procedure

- Do an EUA as described in Section 8.3.
- Determine any other pathology (such as an anal fissure, haemorrhoids etc.) and treat appropriately.
- Inject Bupivicaine with 1:200,000 Epinephrine subcutaneously (and submucosally if needed) under the warts, lifting the wart off the subcutaneous tissue.
- Excise the wart using scissors or a scalpel using a no. 15 blade.
- Smaller warts may be cauterised.

Notes

- Warts may extend into the anal canal; make sure these are treated as well.
- If you are in any way unsure about the diagnosis, send a sample for histological evaluation.

96 Manual of Ambulatory General Surgery

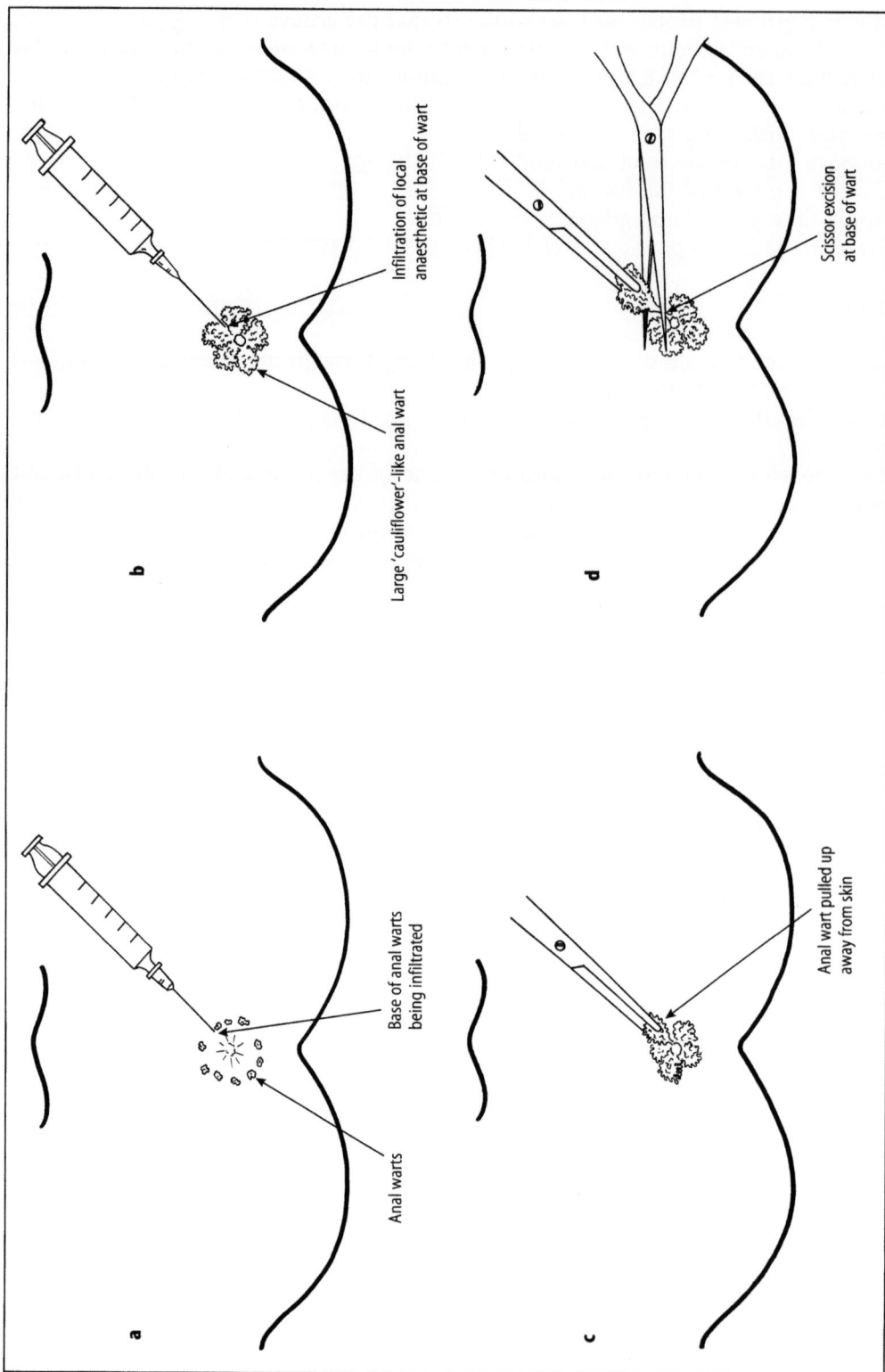

Figure 8.9. Anal warts

- You may need to do the procedure in several sittings if the warts are extensive, in order to avoid anal stenosis post-operatively.
- Ensure that the partner is treated as well.

9 Miscellaneous

9.1 Ganglion

A ganglion is a sac filled with gelatinous material surrounding a tendon sheath. It tends to occur near small joints, commonly on the dorsum of the wrist, but may be found over any joint. It has a high recurrence rate following surgical excision so the patient must be warned of this. On palpation the lump may feel bony hard and may be tender.

Objective   To excise the entire lesion.
Indication   To relieve symptoms of pain/discomfort or for cosmetic reasons.
Setting   Operating theatre/sterile conditions
Preparation   Antiseptic solution.
Anaesthetic   General.
Position   Maximise exposure
                 Place the joint in the neutral position.
                 Use a tourniquet.

Procedure (for a wrist ganglion)

- After the patient is anaesthetised, raise the hand and arm up high for a few minutes in order to empty the veins.
- Apply a tourniquet above the elbow as described in Section 2.2.7 and inflate to above arterial pressure (200 mm Hg usually). Document inflation time.
- Prepare and drape the arm.
- Make the incision over the ganglion, along a skin crease if possible.
- Using scissors, separate the ganglion from the surrounding tissue, creating a plane and dissecting out the ganglion intact.
- Follow the lump down towards the joint or tendon it is attached to, in search of its origin. The aim is to excise as much as possible of the capsule. Take care not to injure tendons in the vicinity (see Figure 9.1).
- Close the skin with interrupted or subcuticular nylon sutures.
- Apply a dry dressing and bandage firmly with a crepe bandage to reduce the chances of a haematoma.
- Deflate the tourniquet and document deflation time (this should be less than 1 hour to be safe).
- Remove sutures after 7 days.

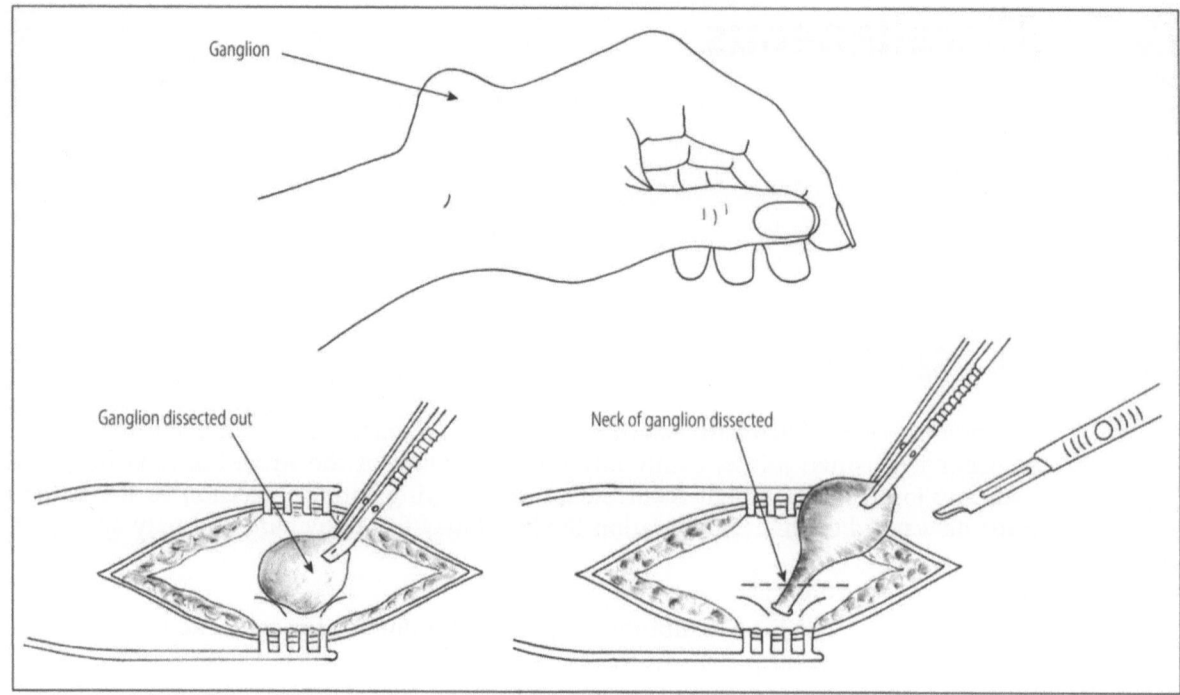

Figure 9.1. Removal of ganglion

9.2 Procedures on Nails

9.2.1 Paronychia

This is a collection of pus at the base of the nail. It should be treated as an abscess, with lancing of the skin to release the pus (also see Section 5.9).

Objective   To release the collection of pus and thus relieve pain.
Indication   Pain and generalised symptoms if unwell.
Setting   Aseptic technique.
Anaesthetic   Digital ring block – do not use Epinephrine (adrenaline).
Preparation   Cleanse the skin with antiseptic solution.
Position   Place the hand on a flat surface.

Procedure

- Make a small stab incision on the summit of the abscess to allow the pus to drain out.
- Squeeze out all the pus.
- Clean the cavity with a syringe of normal saline.
- Cover with a dry dressing.

9.2.2 Subungual Haematoma

This occurs when trauma to the fingernails produces a collection of blood just under the nail. This causes an increase in pressure and can be very painful. Patients complain of a "throbbing" sensation.

The treatment is to release the blood by a trephine of the nail. It should be done within 24 hours of the injury when the blood is still "fluid" and can therefore exude. A longer interval allows the blood to clot and re-organise and will not then flow out.

Objective	To release the haematoma.
Indication	Pain.
Setting	Aseptic technique.
Anaesthetic	None required.
Preparation	Cleanse the finger with antiseptic solution, for example iodine or chlorhexidine.
Position	Place the hand firmly on a flat surface.

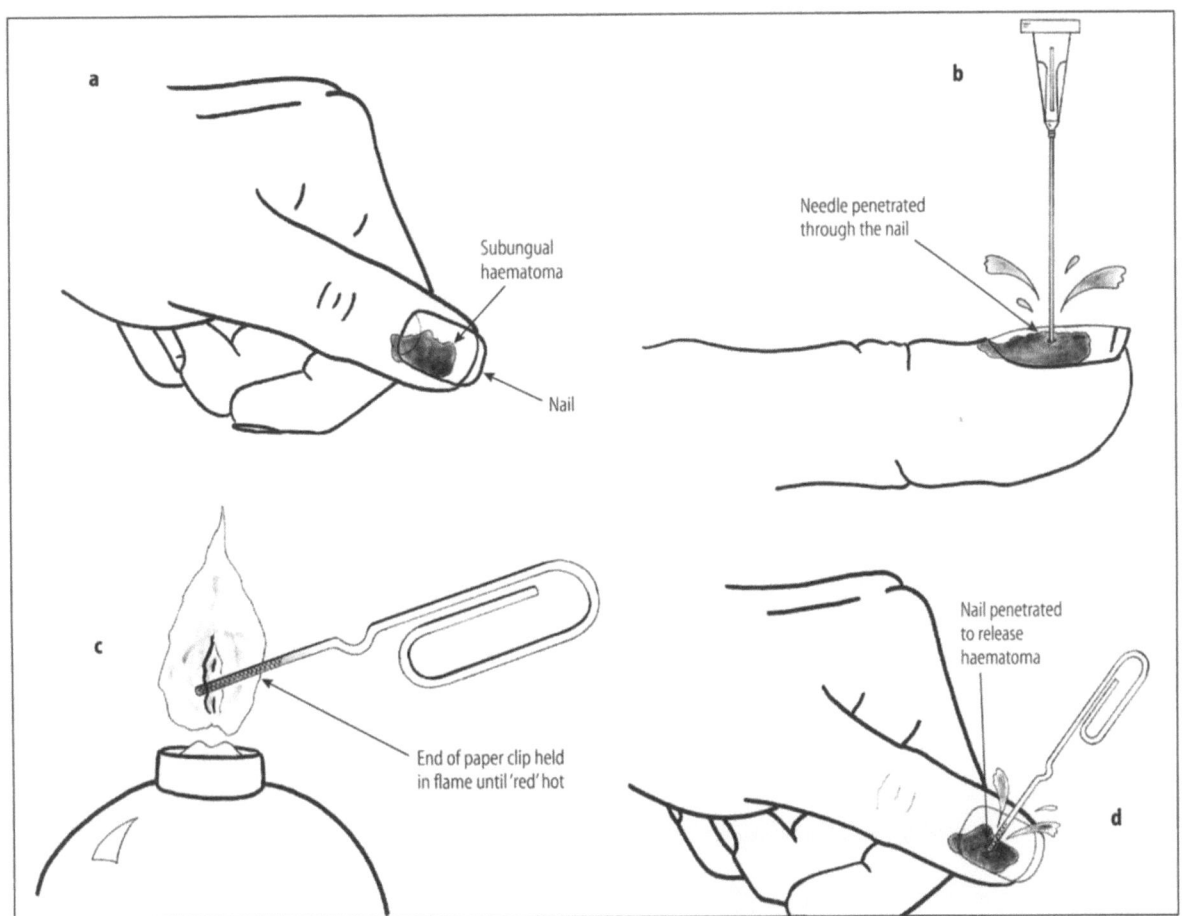

Figure 9.2. Treatment of subungual haematoma

Procedure

- A nail trephine can be done in one of two ways:
  1. Using a 19G needle ("white"), place the point directly onto the nail in the middle of the haematoma. With a rotating action gradually "drill" a hole in the nail. Once the hole is made, the blood will spurt out as it is under pressure. As the needle approaches the nail bed, it may become painful.
  2. Using a stainless steel paper clip, straighten one end. Heat this end in a flame (for example methylated spirit wick) until it is red hot. Gently touch the nail over the haematoma. The heat burns a hole into the nail, allowing the haematoma to escape. If the nail is very thick and hard, it may be necessary to repeat the procedure until the nail is perforated.
- Cover with a dry dressing.

9.2.3 Simple Avulsion of a Nail

This is performed when access to the nail bed is required, for example to suture a laceration or to obtain a biopsy. It may also be performed to simply remove the nail if it is broken and awkward. It is used by some surgeons as a treatment for ingrowing toenails. However, it has a high recurrence rate.

Objective	To remove the nail.
Indication	Diagnostic or therapeutic.
Setting	Aseptic technique.
Anaesthetic	Digital ring block.
Preparation	Clean the finger and nail thoroughly with antiseptic solution.

Procedure

- Separate the nail from the nail bed by inserting a pair of flat scissors or one limb of a large flat arterial clip between them. Take care not to traumatise the nail bed.
- Use arterial forceps to grasp the nail and avulse it with a twisting action.

9.2.4 Lateral Wedge Excision

Wedge resection of a toenail is performed for ingrowing toenails which become inflamed and infected. The big toe is the most commonly affected, especially the lateral edge.

Objective	To excise the lateral edge of the nail and its nail bed (germinal matrix) as well as the adjacent inflamed area and scar tissue (see Figure 9.3).
Indication	Ingrowing toenail.
Setting	Operating theatre.
Position	Supine.
Preparation	Cleanse the skin thoroughly with iodine solution. Clean the spaces between the toes thoroughly, as these wounds are notorious for post-operative infections.

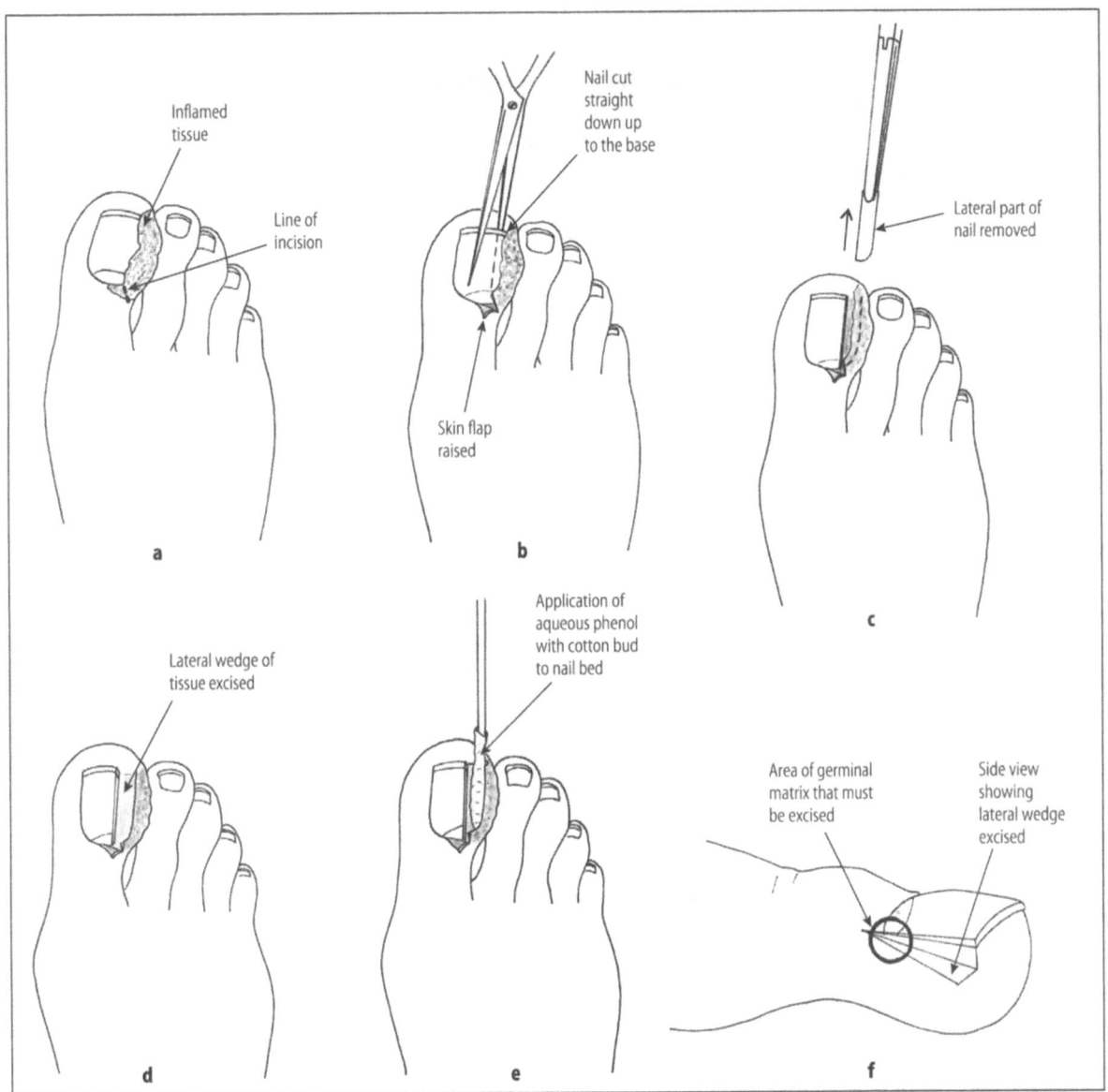

Figure 9.3. Wedge excision of nail

Anaesthetic   Local anaesthetic ring block. Infiltrate the base of the toe with **plain** local anaesthetic, aiming for the digital nerves on either side of the toe. Remember that the digital nerves run along the plantar aspect of the toe. **Do not use Epinephrine (adrenaline).**

Procedure
- Apply a tourniquet to the base of the toe.
- Make a small diagonal incision (about 1 cm) running laterally from the corner of the base of the nail and raise a flap of skin using a scalpel.

- Using a sharp pair of scissors insert one blade under the nail to lift it off the nail bed. Cut the nail straight along the edge removing about 5 mm. Once the entire length of the nail has been divided it is fairly easy to grasp the edge and remove that portion with a rotating action.
- Now excise the nail bed. Using a scalpel, excise the soft tissue, cutting out the lateral edge plus the germinal epithelium. This part of the procedure is the most important, as any residual germinal matrix will result in regrowth of the nail.
- Optional: using a cotton bud dipped in phenol 80 per cent, apply a drop to the nail bed for 1 minute. An immediate blanching effect is seen as cauterisation occurs. Petroleum jelly can be smeared over the adjacent skin to prevent contact. The phenol should then be neutralised with surgical spirit (alcohol) and washed out with normal saline.
- Place Kaltostat or paraffin gauze dressing in the defect.
- Cover with dry gauze wrapped around the toe.
- Apply a 2-inch crepe bandage around the toe fairly tightly, leaving the tip exposed to observe the perfusion.
- Remove the tourniquet.

Post-op. Change the dressing after 24 hours.
Give analgesia as required.

9.2.5 Zadek's Operation

This involves removal of the entire nail and germinal matrix.

Indication Ingrowing toenails – especially those that recur even after wedge excision. It can be performed in the first instance if the patient is not concerned about cosmesis. The usual indication, though, is onychogryphosis.
Objective To remove the whole nail and nail bed.
Setting Operating theatre.
Preparation Cleanse the toe with iodine.
Anaesthetic Digital ring block.

Procedure

- Apply a tourniquet at the base of the toe.
- Raise a skin flap at the base of the nail by making two small incisions extending laterally (see Figure 9.4). Use a scalpel to gently lift the skin off the nail.
- Avulse the nail with artery forceps or a Kocher's instrument. Place one blade under the nail and apply a twisting action.
- The germinal matrix will be visible as white soft tissue. Excise a rectangular area encompassing the entire germinal matrix and ensure that the medial and lateral corners are meticulously removed.
- Optional: cauterise the nail bed with phenol 80 per cent for 1 minute applied with a cotton bud.
- Neutralise the phenol with surgical spirit and then wash out with normal saline.

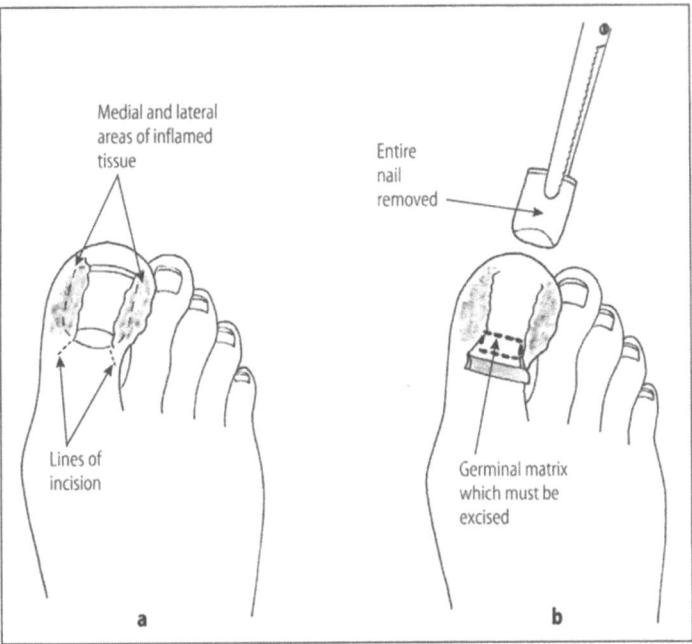

Figure 9.4. Zadek procedure

- Apply Kaltostat or paraffin gauze dressing to the wound.
- Cover with dry gauze and a crepe bandage, leaving the tip exposed to assess the perfusion.
- Release the tourniquet.

Post-op.   Change the dressing after 24 hours.
              Give analgesia as required.

9.3 Muscle Biopsy

This is usually carried out as a diagnostic procedure (for example for rheumatology). Ideally, the most symptomatic muscle should be biopsied. It is important not to biopsy a muscle that has had EMG studies done recently. It is also important not to infiltrate the muscle with local anaesthetic during the procedure and to handle it as little as possible. The histologist may also require you to orientate the biopsy in a particular manner. So before proceeding with this procedure please make sure that you are familiar with the local practice. It is usual to warn the histologist that you are performing the biopsy, as they will have to make special preparations for this. The biopsy is **not** placed in formalin and is sent to the histology department immediately (usually placed on a piece of blotting paper).

Objective   To obtain a good-sized "representative" sample of muscle.
Indication   Diagnostic, for example, polymyalgia rheumatica.
Setting   Operating theatre/sterile conditions.

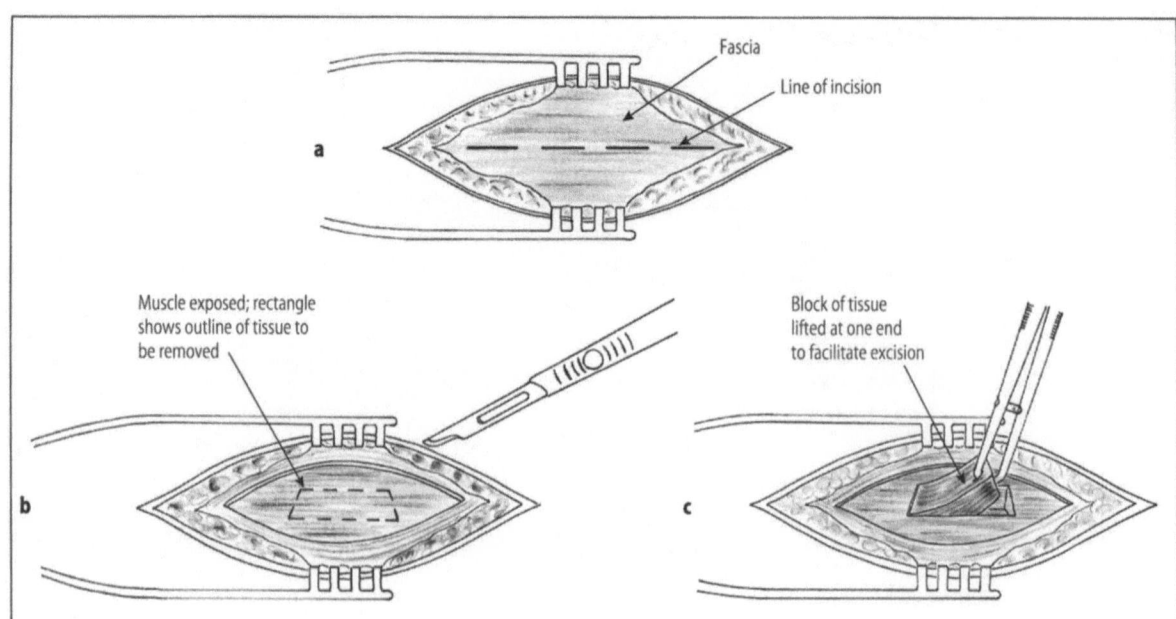

Figure 9.5. Muscle biopsy

Position   Expose the area.
Place the patient in a comfortable position.

Anaesthetic   Local.
This is to be used on the skin and subcutaneous tissue only. It is important **not** to infiltrate the muscle as this interferes with the histology. Inform the patient therefore that the removal of the muscle itself may be painful.

Procedure

- Cleanse the skin with iodine.
- Make an incision (about 5 cm) directly overlying the muscle to be biopsied. Using scissors, dissect away the subcutaneous fat to expose fascia and muscle.
- Insert a self-retaining retractor to keep the wound open.
- Use a scalpel to incise the fascia. Cut out a rectangular block of muscle of approximately 1 cm × 0.5 cm × 0.5 cm.
- Ensure haemostasis.
- Lay the tissue longitudinally on a piece of paper to orientate the fibres for the pathologist.
- There is no need to close the defect in the muscle.
- Close the fascia over the muscle with absorbable sutures such as 3/0 Vicryl
- Close the skin with interrupted or subcuticular sutures (for example 3/0 Prolene or 4/0 PDS.

Post-op.   Remove sutures after 10 days

9.4 Temporal Artery Biopsy

This is carried out for the diagnosis of temporal arteritis or polymyalgia rheumatica.

Objective   To obtain a small segment (1 to 1.5 cm) of the temporal artery for pathological examination.
Indication   Diagnostic.
Setting   Operating theatre/sterile conditions.
Position   Take the biopsy from the side that is most symptomatic. If there is no lateralisation of symptoms, then either temporal artery will do. Lay the patient down with the head turned away from you, exposing the side of the face adequately. Palpate the artery and determine its course along the temple, usually just in front of the hairline (some surgeons prefer to biopsy the segment of the artery just in front of the ear). Mark on the skin a 1 to 2 cm segment of the artery along its course. Sometimes the artery is not pulsatile but is palpable as a thin cord. In difficult cases, a hand-held Doppler can be used to detect the pulsation and map the artery.
Anaesthetic   Local.

Procedure

- Make a 2 cm incision 1 mm alongside the artery to avoid cutting into it.
- Use a self-retaining retractor or skin hooks to hold the wound open.
- Expose the artery with gentle dissection using scissors and artery forceps. The artery lies above the fascia.

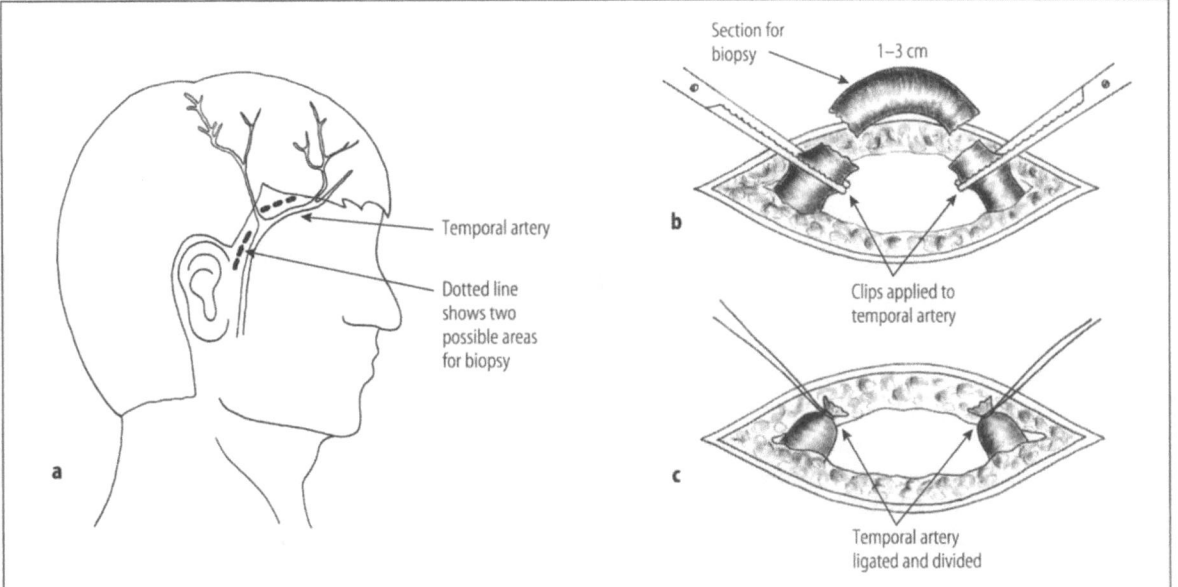

Figure 9.6.   Temporal artery biopsy

- The artery should be seen pulsating.
- Place two haemostats at either end of the exposed segment about 1.5 cm apart. Divide the artery obtaining a small segment.
- If you are in doubt about whether you have really biopsied the artery, temporarily release the proximal clip to ensure the bleeding is pulsatile. Take care that the artery does not retract out of site, as this may result in a haematoma. Re-apply the clip.
- Ligate the ends with 3/0 Vicryl. Send the sample in formalin for histology.
- Ensure haemostasis.
- Close the skin with 5/0 PDS subcuticular or 5/0 Prolene interrupted sutures.
- Spray the wound with op-site dressing.

Post-op. Remove the sutures after 5 days.

9.5 Amputation of a Toe

Amputation of a toe or part of a toe is performed for gangrene usually due to peripheral vascular disease or diabetes mellitus. It is also performed for deformed toes if causing pain. It is important that a vascular work-up has been undertaken prior to toe amputations and that any vascular reconstructive surgery needed is done first.

Objective To remove the affected part of the toe.
Indication Infection and/or pain.
Setting Operating theatre/sterile conditions.
Position Supine with leg extended.
Anaesthetic General, regional or local.

Procedure

- The skin incision must be made distal to the joint being disarticulated in order to obtain loose skin cover. Equal or unequal anterior and posterior flaps may be used, depending on the situation.
- Equal flaps: make a transverse curved incision on the dorsal and plantar aspects of the toe to form equal anterior and posterior flaps (see Figure 9.7).
- Unequal flaps: make a linear transverse incision anteriorly just beyond the level of disarticulation and a generous curved incision posteriorly in order to obtain skin cover after the amputation (see Figure 9.7).
- Divide the tissues down to bone.
- If close to a joint, for example metatarsophalangeal or interphalangeal, aim to disarticulate at the joint. Otherwise use a bone cutter to divide the bone and then a bone nibbler to remove the sharp edges or spikes of bone.
- Pull the exposed tendons and cut back as far as possible, allowing them to retract.
- Close the skin with interrupted 3/0 Prolene sutures.
- Apply gauze and dry dressing.

Post-op. Remove the sutures after 14 days.

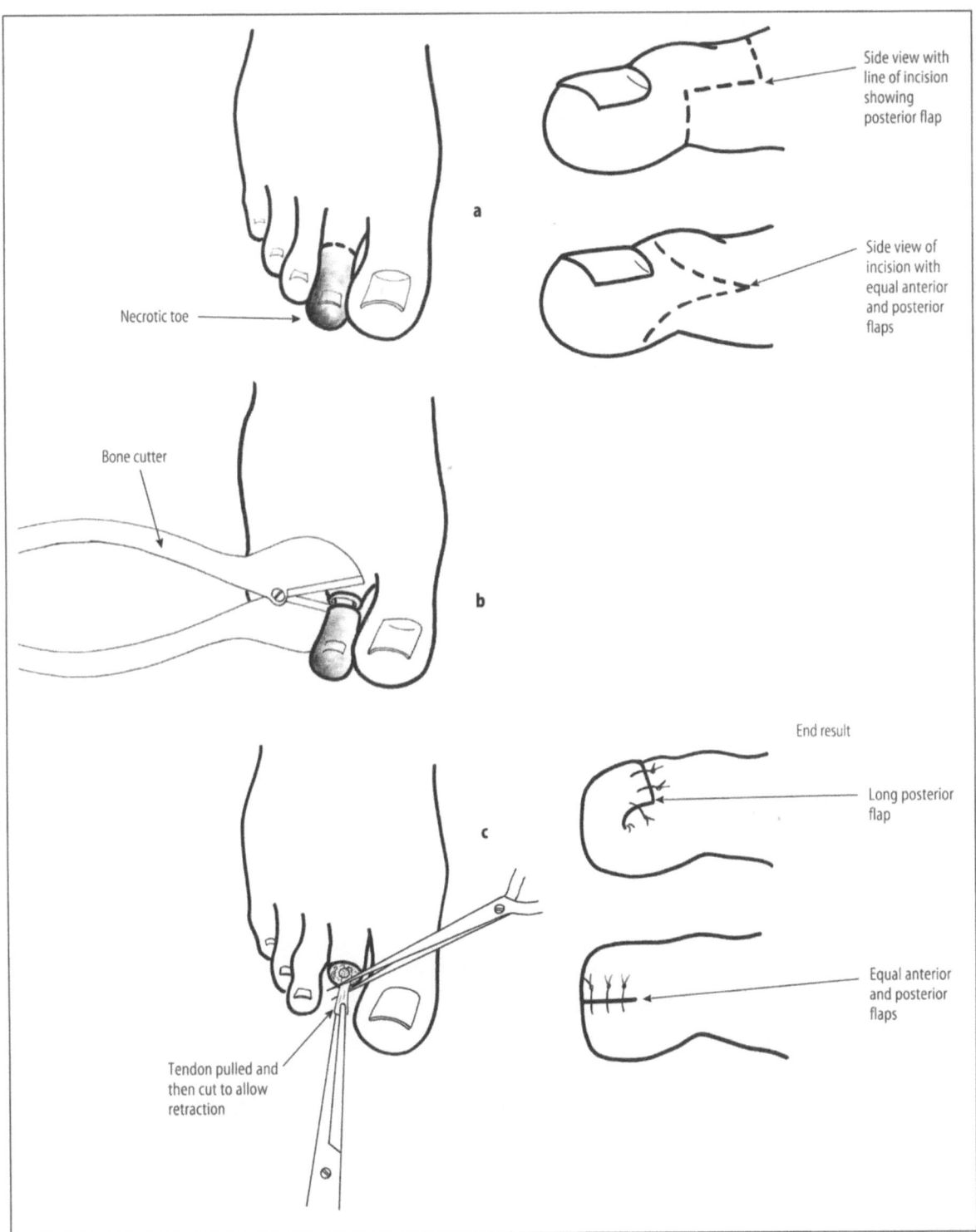

Figure 9.7. Amputation of toe

9.6 Catheterisation

Catheterisation is performed to drain the bladder of urine, either to relieve obstruction beyond the bladder, to drain urine in a bedridden patient or to monitor the output of urine. Most of the time it is done through a urethral catheter. However, in some circumstances a suprapubic catheter is needed.

9.6.1 Urethral Catheterisation

Catheterisation of the urethra is performed

- to relieve urinary retention
- to monitor urine output and renal function
- prior to pelvic or abdominal surgery
- prior to major surgery
- in a bedridden patient.

There is a risk of introducing infection via the breached urethral mucosa, usually gram-negative rods such as E. Coli or Proteus. It should therefore be done gently and with great care. In general, antibiotics are not given to cover this procedure unless specifically indicated.

There are several types of catheters available, made of different materials and varying in size. A Foley catheter is suitable for short-term use, whereas a Silastic catheter is more rigid and would be more suitable for long-term use. The size is denoted by French gauge (F), from 12F which is of a small circumference, to 20F, which has a large circumference. On average, the 14F catheter is ideal.

It is important to set up a trolley with everything you require before you start. Ensure there is a second person with you in case you require further help.

The procedure is performed using aseptic technique with sterile equipment.

Items required   draping sheet
gloves
plastic forceps
gauze
chlorhexidine solution and container
lubricant containing anaesthetic, for example Lidocaine gel
catheter in covering plastic sleeve
kidney dish
syringe containing 10 to 30 ml sterile water (depending on balloon size of catheter)
drainage bag with connecting tube.

Anaesthetic   Gel containing local anaesthetic.

Position   Supine with legs spread apart. This is essential in females and better exposure is obtained with flexion of the knees, and abduction with external rotation of the hips.

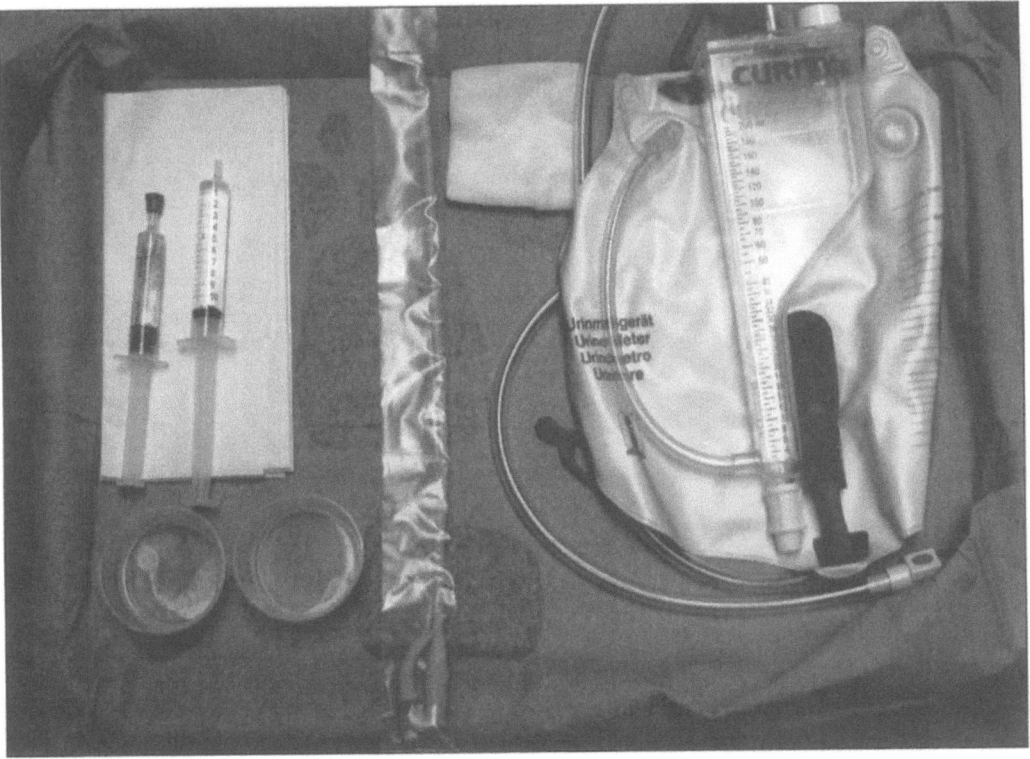

Figure 9.8. Items required for catheterisation

Procedure

- Put on sterile gloves.
- Prepare your trolley so that you have easy access to all the items.
- Place the draping sheet over the lower abdomen and legs with a hole in the middle of the sheet to expose only enough area to gain access to the urethra.
- Designate the left hand as your "dirty" hand and the right hand as the "clean" hand. This means that the left hand will come into contact with the patient and the right hand will be used to handle the catheter.
- Use plastic forceps and gauze soaked in chlorhexidine to clean the area thoroughly.

In the female

- Using forceps and gauze soaked in antiseptic solution, start off by cleaning the labia, then use the left hand to separate the labia and the right hand to clean the urethral opening and surrounding area. Go from anterior to posterior.
- Split the plastic cover of the catheter along the perforations to expose 5 to 10 cm of the end. Lubricate this end. Hold the catheter covered with its sleeve and introduce the tip into the urethra up to the sleeve. Then pull the sleeve back a further 5 to 10 cm and advance the catheter. Repeat this until urine flows out. Use a kidney dish to receive the urine and avoid spillage. See Figure 9.9.
- Now dilate the balloon with the required amount of water, usually 10 ml (the amount needed will be written on the catheter).

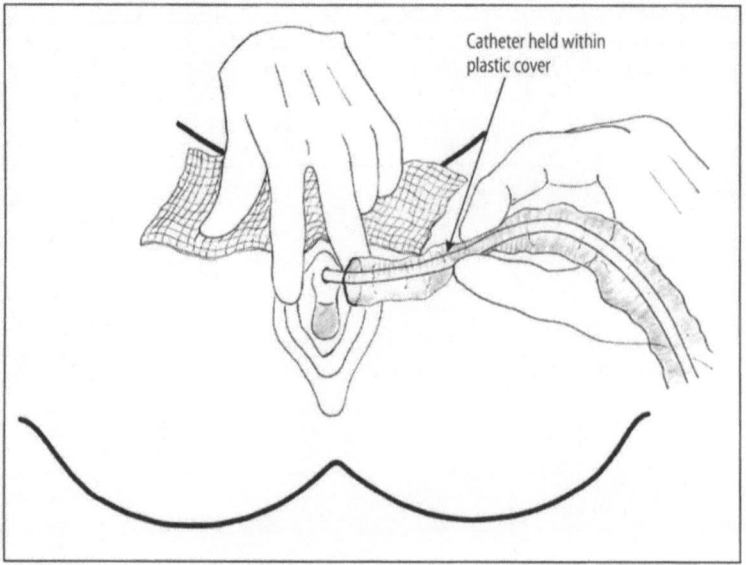

Figure 9.9. Female catheterisation

- Connect the drainage bag tubing to the catheter.
- Pull the catheter back gently to check it is secure. Then push the catheter into the bladder a slight amount so that it is left sitting loosely, thus avoiding bladder neck necrosis.

In the male

- Use the left hand to hold the penis covered with gauze, clean thoroughly, retract the foreskin if present, and clean the urethral meatus.
- Instil the lubricant gel into the urethra. Gently squeeze the tip of the penis to contain the gel.
- Split the plastic cover of the catheter along the perforations to expose 5 to 10 cm of the end.
- Hold the catheter covered with its sleeve and introduce the tip into the urethra up to the sleeve. Then pull the sleeve back a further 5 to 10 cm and advance the catheter. Repeat this until urine flows out. Use a kidney dish to receive the urine and avoid spillage.
- Now dilate the balloon with the required amount of water, usually 10 to 30 ml. Check the amount required on the individual catheter.
- Connect the drainage bag tubing to the catheter.
- Pull the catheter back gently to check it is secure. Then push the catheter into the bladder a slight amount so that it is left sitting loosely, thus avoiding bladder neck necrosis.
- Pull back the foreskin (in the uncircumcised male) to avoid a paraphimosis developing.

To remove the catheter, again use aseptic technique. Deflate the balloon and pull the catheter out gently.

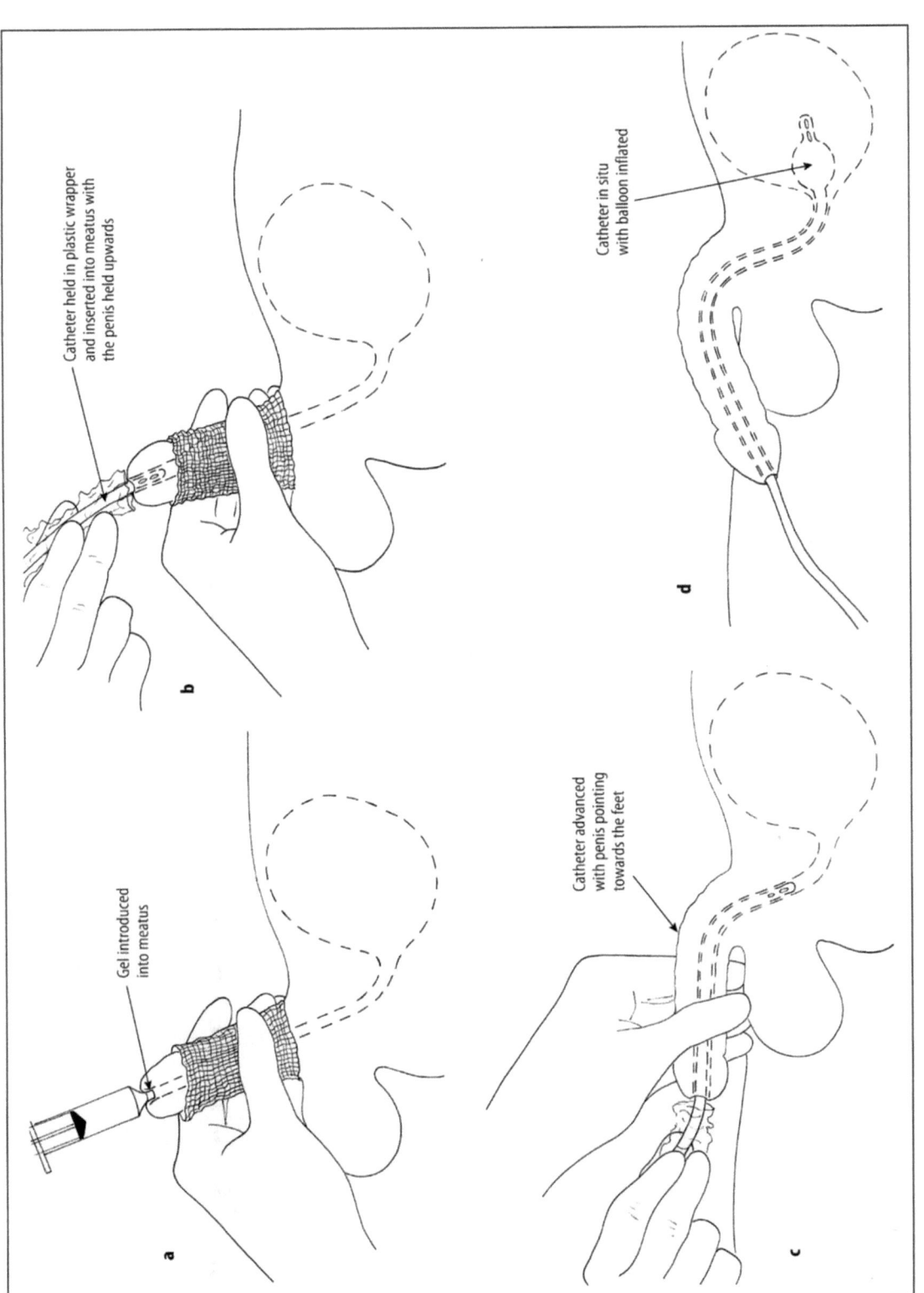

Figure 9.10. Male catheterisation

114 Manual of Ambulatory General Surgery

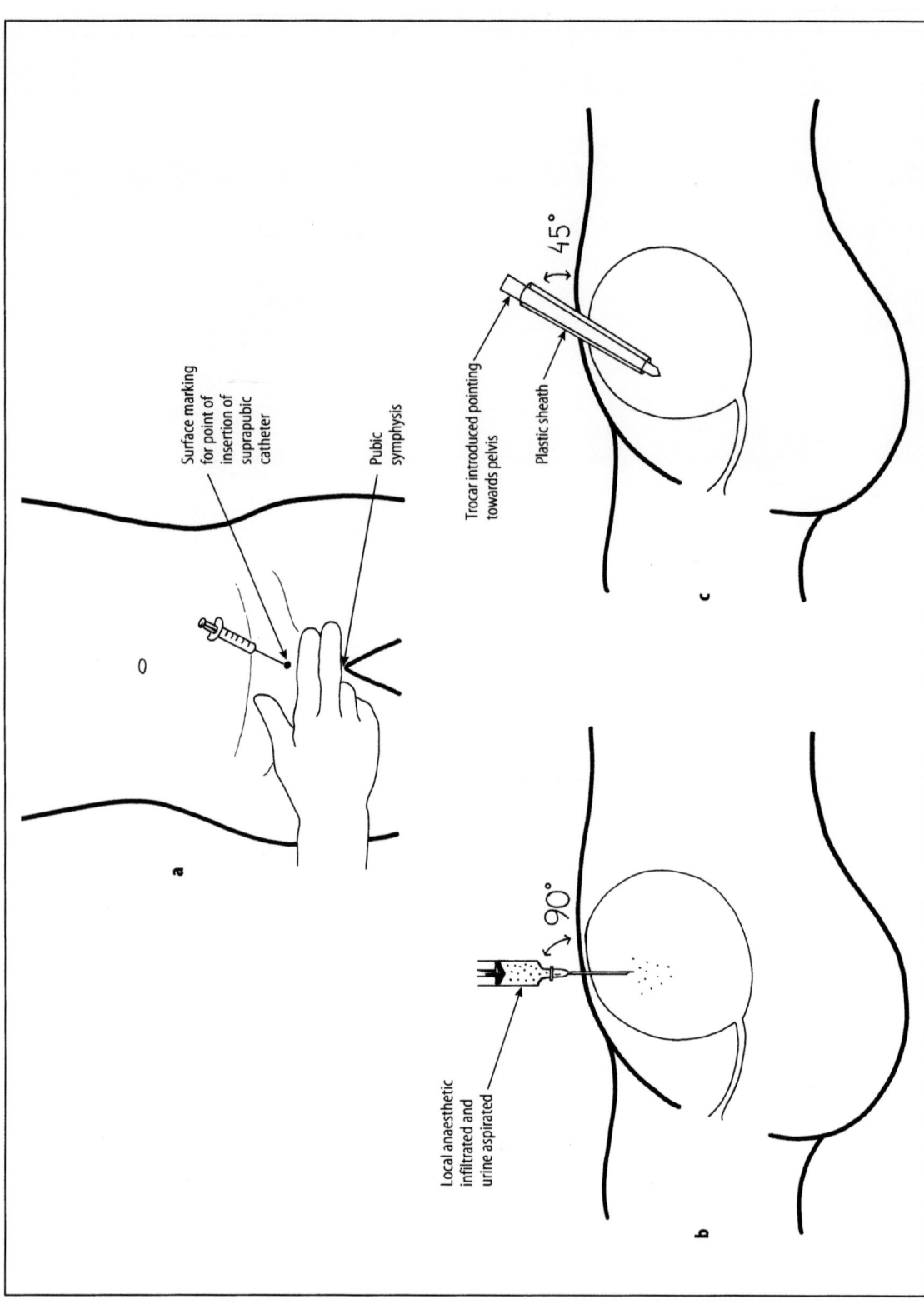

Figure 9.11. Suprapubic catheterisation

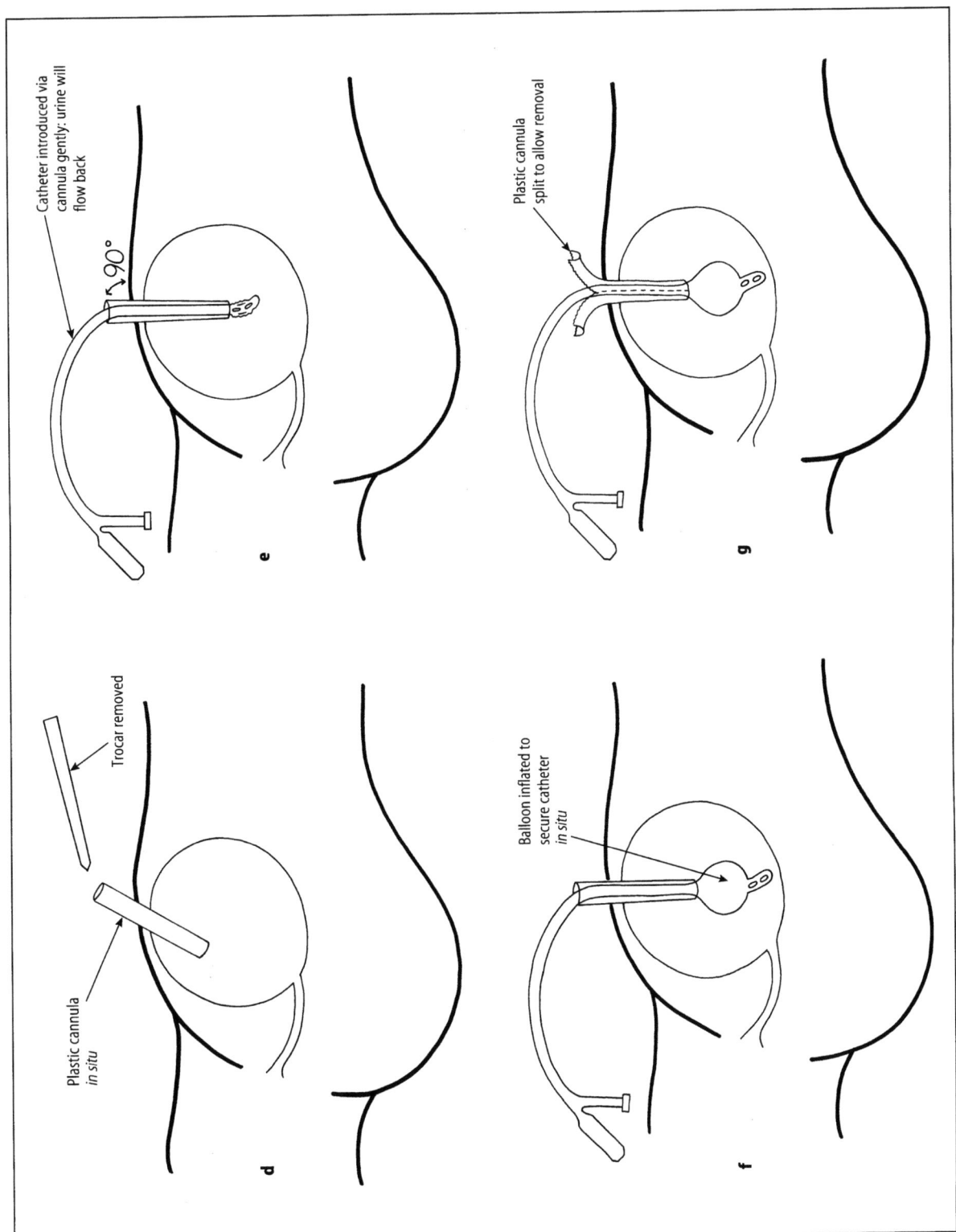

9.6.2 Suprapubic Catheterisation

Suprapubic catheterisation is performed in instances when urethral catheterisation is not feasible, for example, urethral obstruction or urethral trauma.

It should be done with a full bladder and you should percuss the bladder to check this. The surface marking for the point of insertion of the trocar (and catheter) is 3 to 4 cm (or two fingerbreadths) above the symphysis pubis in the midline.

Setting	Aseptic technique/operating theatre.
Position	Supine. Expose the abdomen from the umbilicus to the groin.
Preparation	Cleanse the skin with antiseptic solution.
	Drape the area with the suprapubic region exposed adequately.
Anaesthesia	Local. Use 5 ml of local anaesthetic to infiltrate the skin and subcutaneous tissue in the suprapubic area 3 cm above the pubis.
	At this point it is worth inserting your needle into the bladder and aspirating urine to confirm the position of the bladder directly beneath the entry point.

Procedure

- Make a small 5 mm incision in the skin over the point of entry of the needle.
- Use the index finger as a guard alongside the trocar to maintain control and avoid slipping as you advance it. Insert the trocar and covering sheath through the small incision with the trocar pointing towards the feet at an angle of about 45 degrees to the abdominal wall. Use a twisting action to pierce the abdominal wall and then the bladder. Once the bladder wall is penetrated, urine will flow up the sheath.
- Remove the trocar.
- Insert the catheter (a Foley catheter 14F is ideal) through the sheath into the bladder. Check that urine is flowing out of the catheter.
- If the catheter has a balloon, dilate it with the required amount of water, usually 10 ml.
- Connect the drainage bag tubing to the catheter.
- Pull the catheter back gently to check it is secure.
- Remove the sheath by splitting it at the groove along its length.
- You may wish to secure the catheter to the skin using a non-absorbable suture such as 2/0 silk. However, this is not essential if the catheter has a balloon, as the balloon will stop the catheter from "falling out".
- To remove the catheter, use aseptic technique. Deflate the balloon and withdraw the catheter gently.

9.7 Circumcision

Circumcision is the excision of the penile foreskin. It is done for various reasons at different ages. In babies, it is usually done for religious reasons. In children there are two main problems that warrant circumcision: recurrent balanitis with severe infections and a tight foreskin where the urethral meatus is obscured, usually causing ballooning of the foreskin during urination. In most children, minor symptoms tend to resolve, but in more persistent cases it should be dealt with. Circumcision may be performed in adults for recurrent infections, paraphimosis or on request.

9.7.1 Conventional Technique (suitable for children and adults)

Objective   To excise the penile foreskin.
Indication Recurrent balanitis, phimosis, paraphimosis, social and religious reasons.
Setting   Operating theatre, sterile conditions. Do not use monopolar diathermy under any circumstances, as this may cause thrombosis of the whole of the corpus cavernosum. Bipolar diathermy is permissible; however, we recommend the procedure is done without the use of diathermy altogether.
Position   Supine.
Anaesthetic General.

Procedure

- Separate the foreskin from the glans penis. Do this by retracting the foreskin and gently separating it from the glans with a pledget and/or arterial forceps, using an opening action.
- Clean the glans penis and coronal sulcus with antiseptic solution.
- Pull the foreskin back over the glans. Place a straight haemostat along the midline of the dorsal surface of the foreskin.
- Crush the foreskin up to 5 mm from the coronal sulcus. See Figure 9.12.
- Use a pair of scissors to incise the foreskin straight through the middle of the crushed area, thus splitting the foreskin into two "halves".
- Grasp the foreskin with two arterial forceps, one placed on each corner of the cut edges.
- Place two further arterial forceps on each cut edge just next to the apex of the cut.
- Keeping the foreskin taut (by having an assistant pull on the arterial forceps on one half of the foreskin), use scissors to cut through the skin circumferentially and parallel to the coronal sulcus, about 5 mm away from it. As you approach the midline on the ventral surface, form a peak to accommodate the frenulum and stop there. Now cut the other "half" of the foreskin starting at the apex of your initial cut and working towards the frenulum.
- Clip and ligate the frenular artery with 3/0 catgut or Vicryl.
- Pick up any other bleeding points with arterial forceps ("mosquito") and ligate.
- Suture the skin and deeper mucosal edge together with interrupted 3/0 catgut or Vicryl.
- Cover with paraffin gauze and a dry dressing, leaving the meatus exposed for the passage of urine.

Post-op.   Observe the wound for bleeding.
             The dressing can be removed after 24 hours.
             Expect some oedema and swelling which should settle after 3 or 4 days

118 Manual of Ambulatory General Surgery

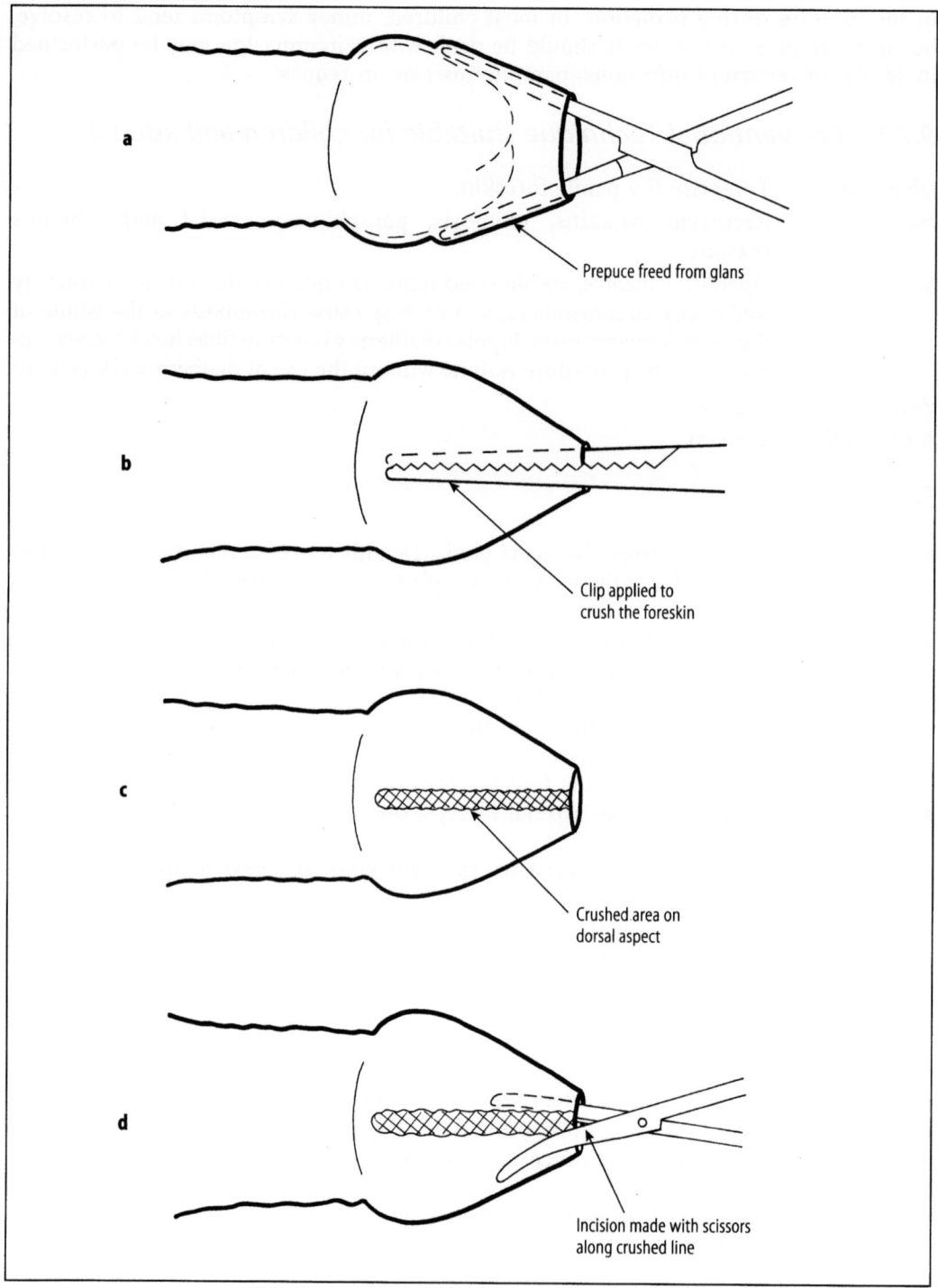

Figure 9.12. Circumcision: conventional technique

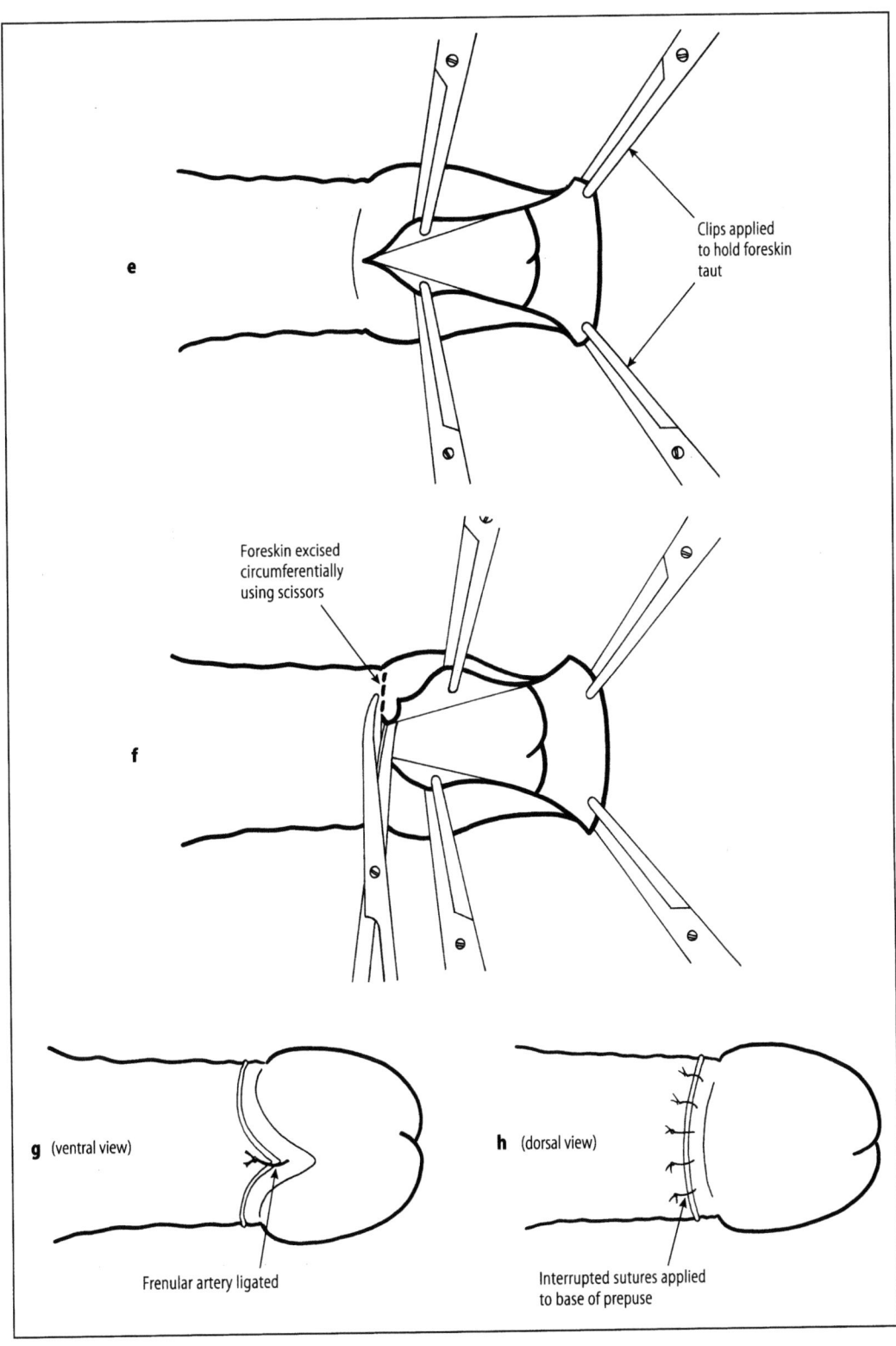

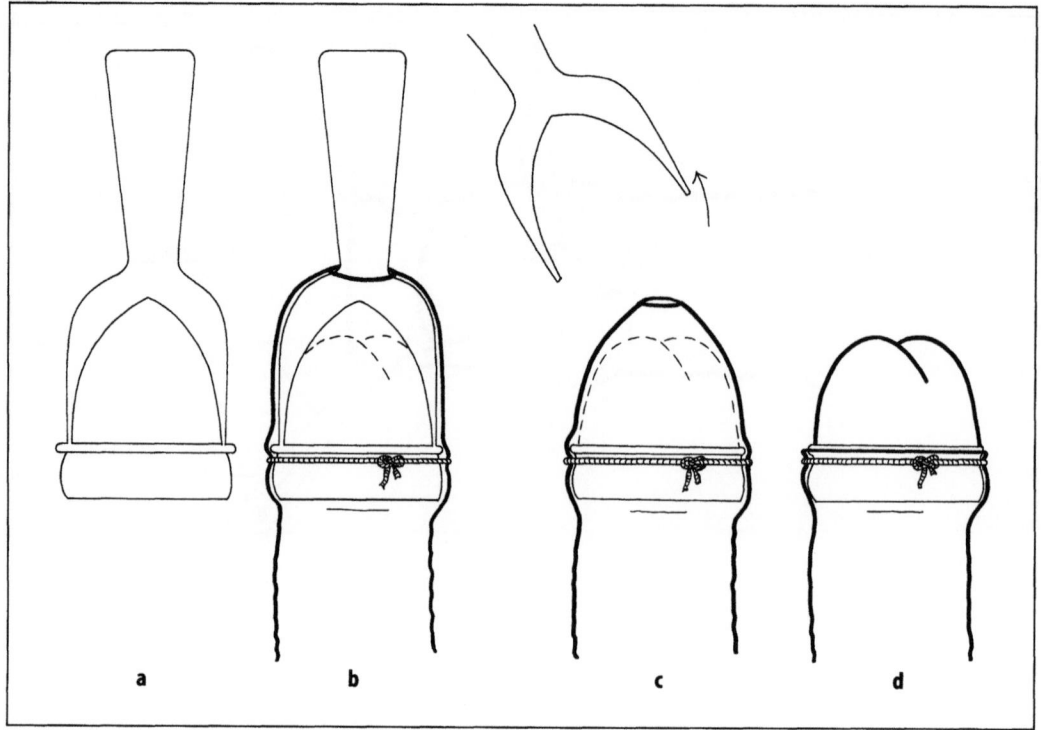

Figure 9.13 Circumcision: Plastibell technique

9.7.2 Plastibell Technique (suitable for infants)

Used in neonates, this is a plastic bell-like contraption. It is placed between the glans and foreskin. A ligature is then tied in position tightly around the bell (see Figure 9.13) in a groove about 5 mm from the coronal sulcus. The foreskin is excised with scissors and the handle is then snapped off. Any skin beyond the ligature undergoes necrosis and separates. The remainder heals well.

9.8 Vasectomy

Vasectomy is used as a method of contraception. Patients should receive counselling and be given accurate information before the procedure is performed. It may be useful to talk to both partners. The following points should be covered:

- The patient's family should be complete and no further children wanted.
- Details of the operation should be explained and that it can be performed under local or general anaesthesia.
- Attempts at reversing the procedure have a significant failure rate and therefore a vasectomy should be considered to be irreversible.

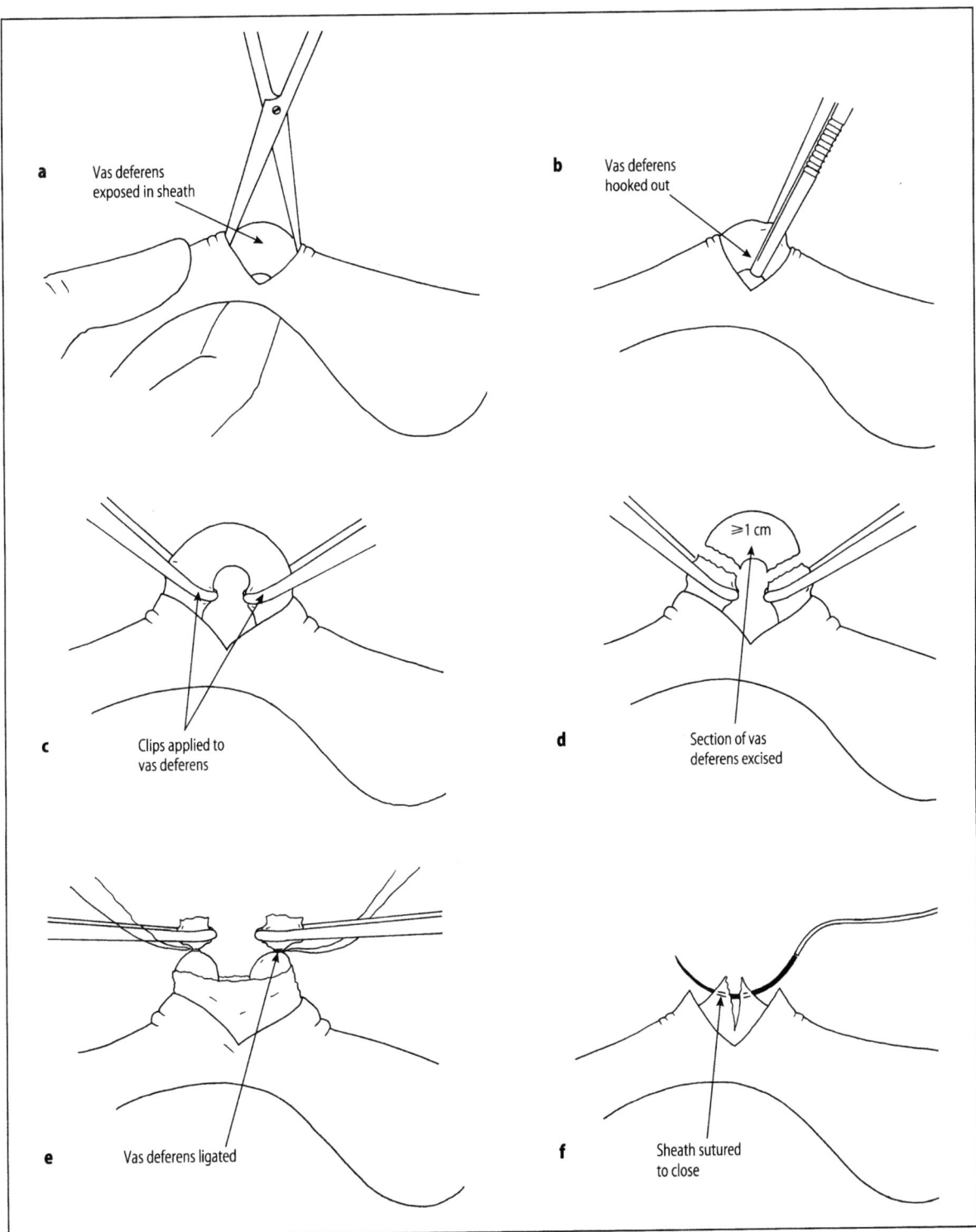

Figure 9.14 Vasectomy

- The operation may fail, and other forms of contraception are needed until two consecutive sperm tests are negative and histological examination of the specimens sent confirms that both sections removed were vas deferens.

Objective Male sterilisation by means of cutting a section out of each vas deferens (vas) and tying the cut ends securely.
Indications Male sterilisation.
Setting Operating theatre.
Position Supine.
Anaesthetic Local or general.

Procedure

- Palpate the vas on one side between thumb and index finger above the testes high up in the scrotum.
- Place the vas as subcutaneous as possible by rolling it under the skin with one hand and then grasping it with another.
- If using local anaesthetic, hold the vas firmly in its subcutaneous placement and infiltrate the skin overlying it with local anaesthetic.
- Keeping your index finger and thumb just behind and on either side of the vas to keep it in place, make an incision in the scrotal skin in line with the underlying vas using a scalpel with a no. 15 blade mounted on it. Cut down until you can see the vas (there are always more layers than you think).
- It may be necessary to infiltrate the sheath and the vas with local anaesthetic at this point.
- Isolate the vas within its sheath using an Allis forceps (or a vasectomy hook). Dissect the vas out of its sheath to expose 2 cm of its length.
- Confirm that it is the vas by rolling it in your fingers. It should be white in colour and feel hard and cord-like.
- Apply two artery forceps to the vas placing them about 2 cm apart.
- Use a scalpel to divide the vas at each end and remove at least a 1 cm segment.
- Ask for the removed section to be placed in a histology specimen pot and labelled according to the side it was removed from, and send it off for histology.
- Ligate the two ends with 2/0 Vicryl.
- Check for haemostasis.
- Close the dartos fascia with 3/0 Vicryl. Grasping it (immediately under the scrotal skin) on each side with an Allis forceps facilitates suturing it together (use a continuous stitch). The scrotal skin does not need to be closed.
- Spray the wound with op-site spray.
- Do the same on the other side.
- Cover the wounds with a small piece of dry gauze.
- Apply a scrotal support.

Post-op. Inform the patient that he will only be declared sterile once the histology has confirmed that the sections removed are indeed vas **and** when two samples of semen taken at 8 and 12 weeks after the operation have shown that there is no sperm in the semen. Until that time, additional birth control measures must be used.

Appendix A
Scrub and Operative Field Preparation Solutions

Surgical Scrub Solutions

- 7.5 per cent povidone-iodine solution (0.75 per cent w/w available iodine) (Videne).
  Adams Healthcare Leeds LS25 2JY.
- 7.5 per cent povidone-iodine solution (Betadine).
  Zeneca, Macclesfield, Cheshire SK10 4TG.
- 4 per cent chlorhexidine gluconate solution (Hydrex).
  Adams Healthcare Leeds LS25 2JY.
- 4 per cent chlorhexidine gluconate solution (Hibiscrub).
  Zeneca, Macclesfield, Cheshire, SK10 4TG.

Antiseptic Solutions for the Preparation of Operative Sites

- 10 per cent povidone-iodine in **aqueous** solution (1 per cent w/w available iodine) (Videne).
  Adams Healthcare Leeds LS25 2JY.
- 10 per cent povidone-iodine in **aqueous** solution.
  Seton Healthcare Group plc, 0161 652 2222.
- 10 per cent povidone-iodine in **spirit*** (1 per cent w/w available iodine) (Videne).
  Adams Healthcare, Leeds LS25 2JY.
- 10 per cent povidone-iodine in **spirit***.
  Seton Healthcare Group plc, 0161 652 2222.
- pink chlorhexidine gluconate (0.5 per cent w/v in 70 per cent v/v industrial methylated **spirit**)* (Hydrex).
  Adams Healthcare, Leeds LS25 2JY.
- 0.05 per cent aqueous chlorhexidine.
  Seton Healthcare Group plc, 0161 652 2222.

---

*Avoid spirit based solutions on mucous membranes. Do not use spirit based solutions if you do not wish pre-operation skin markings to be rubbed off during preparation (use an aqueous solution instead).

Appendix B
Dosages of Popular Local Anaesthetics, Sedatives and Analgesics used in Local Anaesthetic Operations

Local anaesthetics
In a 70 Kg man the maximum dosages are as follows:

Agent	Maximum dose (mg)*	0.25 per cent solution (ml)	0.5 per cent solution (ml)	1 per cent solution (ml)	2 per cent solution (ml)
Plain Lidocaine (lignocaine)	300	n/a	60	30	15
Lidocaine with 1:200,000 Epinephrine (adrenaline)	500	n/a	100	50	25
Plain Bupivicaine (Marcaine)	175	70	35	17.5	n/a
Bupivicaine with 1:200,000 Epinephrine (adrenaline)	225	90	45	22.5	n/a

*Doses may vary depending on medical conditions. Always consult relevant drug data sheets.

Sedation

Agent	Maximum dose per kg (mg/kg)	Maximum dose in 70 kg man (mg)
Midazolam	0.07 to 0.08	4.9 to 5.6
Diazepam	0.05 to 0.3	3.5 to 21

Analgesia

Agent	Maximum dose per kg (mg/kg)	Maximum dose in 70 kg man (mg)
Pethidine	1 to 1.5	70 to 105

Appendix C
Prophylactic Antibiotic Regimens and Dosages

Always ensure that the patient is not allergic to the antibiotic. The dosages given below relate to an average 70 kg male. Adjustments in dosages need to be made for the age, weight and sex of the patient.

The protocols below are merely guidelines. Some institutions have a local antibiotic policy which may differ from the advice given below.

General Procedure
Broad-spectrum antibiotic such as

- Cefuroxime 1.5 g
- Cephadrine 1 g
- Augmentin 1.2 g
- Amoxycillin 1 g

In patients allergic to penicillins, Erythromycin or Gentamicin may be used. (Remember that 10 per cent of people allergic to penicilllins will also be allergic to cephalosporins.)

Prophylactic antibiotics should be given intravenously just before the incision. (Some surgeons also recommend two further doses at 6 and 12 hours post-operatively.)

Gastro-intestinal Tract Procedures
For gastro-intestinal operations, usually a broad-spectrum antibiotic is given with additional cover against bacteroides (especially in large bowel surgery), for example

- Cefuroxime 1.5 g and Metronidazole 500 mg
- Augmentin 1.2 g

In patients allergic to penicillins, Erythromycin or Gentamicin may be used. (Remember that 10 per cent of people allergic to penicillins will also be allergic to cephalosporins.)

Urological Procedures
Cover against gram-negative oragnisms is needed in urological procedures including removal of catheters. The most commonly used antibiotic for this is

- Gentamicin 80 mg

Vascular Procedures

In patients having vascular procedures, especially amputations, it is important to obtain cover against skin organisms. Commonly used regimens include

- Benzyl penicillin 1.2 g and Flucloxacillin 500 mg
- Amoxycillin 1 g and Flucloxacillin 500 mg
- Cefuroxime 1.5 g and Flucloxacillin 500 mg

If the patient is diabetic, cover against bacteroides is desirable, especially in infected foot surgery. In this case we recommend the addition of Mertonidazole 500 mg to one of the above regimens.

Appendix D
Consent Forms

Consent Form for Investigations, Treatments and Operations

    Hospital . . . .   Patient Number . . . .
    Patient's Surname . . . .   Other Names . . . .
    Date of Birth . . . .   Sex . . . .

This part to be completed by doctor
Name of investigation, treatment or operation: . . . .
. . . .

I confirm that I have explained the investigation, treatment or operation, and such appropriate options as are available to the patient in terms which in my judgement are suited to the understanding of the patient and/or to one of the parents or guardians of the patient.
Signature: . . . .   Date: . . . .
Name of doctor: . . . .

To Patient, Parent or Guardian
1. Please read this form very carefully.
2. If there is anything that you do not understand about the explanation, or if you want more information, you should ask the doctor.
3. Please check that all the information on the form is correct. If it is, and you understand the explanation, then sign the form.

I am the patient/parent/guardian *(delete as necessary)*
I agree
- to what is proposed which has been explained to me by the doctor named on this form.
- to the use of general, regional, local or other anaesthetic as in the opinion of the anaesthetist is appropriate

I understand
- that the procedure may not be done by the doctor who has been treating me so far.
- that any procedure in addition to the investigation or treatment described on this form will only be carried out if it is necessary and in my best interests and can be justified for medical reasons.

I have told the doctor
- the procedures listed below which I would **not** wish to be carried out straightaway without my having the opportunity to consider them first.

. . . .
. . . .

Signature: . . . .   Name: . . . .
Address: . . . .

Example of a typical consent form

Consent Form for Sterilisation or Vasectomy

Hospital .... Patient Number ....
Patient's Surname .... Other Names ....
Date of Birth .... Sex ....

This part to be completed by doctor
Name of operation: STERILISATION/VASECTOMY (Delete as appropriate)

I confirm that I have explained the investigation, treatment or operation, and such appropriate options as are available to the patient in terms which in my judgement are suited to the understanding of the patient and/or to one of the parents or guardians of the patient.
Signature: .... Date: ....
Name of doctor: ....

To Patient
1. Please read this form very carefully.
2. If there is anything that you don't understand about the explanation, or if you want more information, you should ask the doctor.
3. Please check that all the information on the form is correct. If it is, and you understand the explanation, then sign the form.

I am the patient
I agree
- to what is proposed which has been explained to me by the doctor named on this form.
- to the use of general, regional, local or other anaesthetic as in the opinion of the anaesthetist is appropriate

I understand
- that the procedure may not be done by the doctor who has been treating me so far.
- that the aim of the operation is to stop me having any children and it might not be possible to reverse the effects of the operation.
- that sterilisation/vasectomy can sometimes fail, and that there is a very small chance that I may become fertile again after some time.
- that any procedure in addition to the investigation or treatment described on this form will only be carried out if it is necessary and in my best interests and can be justified for medical reasons.

I have told the doctor
- the procedures listed below which I would **not** wish to be carried out straightaway without my having the opportunity to consider them first.

For Vasectomy I understand
- that I may remain fertile or become fertile again after some time.
- that I will have to use some other contraceptive method until two consecutive tests show that I am not producing sperm, if I do not want to father any children.

Signature: .... Name: ....
Address: ....
....

Example of a typical consent for vasectomy or sterilisation

Appendix E
Medical Defence Organisations in the UK

Medical Defence Union

Address	Medical Defence Union Limited
	3 Devonshire Place
	London W1N 2EA
	Telephone: 0171 486 6181 – 0800 716 376
	Fax: 0171 935 5503
	or
	Medical Defence Union Limited
	192 Altrincham Road
	Manchester M22 4RZ
	UK
	Telephone: 0161 428 1234 – 0800 716 376
	Fax: 0161 491 3301 – 0161 491 1420
E-mail	Membership@the-mdu.com
Website	http://www.the-mdu.com

Medical Protection Society

Address	Medical Protection Society
	Granary Wharf House
	Leeds LS11 5PY
	UK
	Telephone: 0345 187187
	Fax: 0113 241 0500
E-mail	Info@mps.org.uk
Website	http://www.mps.org.uk

Index

A
abscess   43–4
adhesive strips   35, 37
amputation, toe   108–9
anaerobic organisms (debridement)   36
anaesthesia
   local   21–5
   nerve block   25
   ring block   24–5
anal
   carcinoma   85
   fissure   85, 88–92
   proctoscopy   81–2
   sigmoidoscopy   82–4
   stretch   89–90
   warts   95–7
anal procedures
   colitis   84
   Crohn's disease   90
   diverticular disease   84
   fistula-in-ano   92–5
   Goodsall's law   92
   lateral (internal) sphincterotomy   90–2
   lithotomy position   81
   Seton procedure   95
analgesics   21
antibiotic prophylaxis   3–5
artery biopsy, temporal   107–8
avulsion, nail   102

B
banding haemorrhoids   86–7
basal cell carcinoma   44–5
biopsy
   muscle   105–6
   skin   49
   temporal artery   107–8
blades, scalpel   9–10
Bowen's disease   50
Bupivicaine   22, 23, 24

C
carcinoma
   anal   85
   basal cell   44–5
   Bowen's disease   50
   malignant melanoma   45–7
   squamous cell   45
catheterisation
   suprapubic   116
   urethral   110–15
central line (vascular access)   27, 28–32
chlorhexidine solution   1
circumcision   116–20
   plastibell technique   120
clips, wound   18–19
colitis, anal procedures   84
consent, patient   6–7
   Hepatitis/HIV testing   6
   operations   6–7
Crohn's disease, anal procedures   90
curettage/curettes   12, 42
cyanoacrylate glue   36–7
cyst
   dermoid   39
   sebaceous   38–9

D
debridement, wound   35–6
dermoid cyst   39

diathermy 19–20
dirty wounds 4, 36
disinfecting, skin 3
diverticular disease, anal procedures 84
Doppler, hand-held (varicose veins) 51, 59
Duplex scanning (varicose veins) 51
   sapheno-popliteal junction 59

E
Epinephrine 21–2, 23, 24

F
femoral hernia 76–7
fissure, anal 85, 88–92
fistula-in-ano, anal procedures 92–5
forcep types 10–11

G
ganglion 99
glue, tissue 35, 36–7
Goodsall's law, anal procedures 92

H
haemorrhoids 85–7
   banding 86–7
hand knotting 17, 19
hand-held Doppler (varicose veins) 51, 59
   sapheno-popliteal junction 59
hepatitis
   protection 5–6
   testing 6
Hepatitis B virus, immunisation 7
hernia
   femoral 76–7
   inguinal 69–76
   para-umbilical 77–9
HIV
   protection 5–6
   testing 6
hydrogen peroxide (debridement) 36
hypertrophic scar 42

I
immunisation, Hepatitis B virus 7
indemnity, medical 6–7
infection, wound 3–5
inguinal hernia 69–76
instrument knotting 17, 19
insurance, malpractice 6–7
internal jugular vein access 31–2
inversion stripping, varicose veins 64–5

J
jugular vein access, internal 31–2

K
keloid scar 42–3
keratosis, solar 50
knots 17–19

L
lacerations
   pretibial 37
   skin 35–7
lateral (internal) sphincterotomy, anal procedures 90–2
Lidocaine 21
lines
   central (vascular access) 27, 28–32
   tunnelled venous 32–3
lipoma 40–1
lithotomy position, anal procedures 81
local anaesthesia 21–5
long saphenous vein (vascular access) 28

M
malignant melanoma 45–7
malpractice insurance 6–7
Mayo repair, para-umbilical hernia 78–9
medical indemnity 6–7
melanoma, malignant 45–7

mesh, polypropylene (inguinal hernia) 74–5
muscle biopsy 105–6

N
naevus, pigmented 41–2
nail bed 102, 103
nails
   avulsion 102
   paronychia 100
   subungual haematoma 101–2
   wedge excision 102–4
   Zadek's operation 104–5
needle holders 10–11
nerve block anaesthesia 25

O
operation note 7–8

P
papilloma 37–8
para-umbilical hernia 77–9
paronychia, nail 100
patient consent 6–7
   Hepatitis/HIV testing 6
   operations 6–7
phlebectomies, varicose veins 65–7
pigmented naevus 41–2
pin stripper, varicose veins 64–5
pinch skin graft 47–8
plastibell technique, circumcision 120
polypropylene mesh (inguinal hernia) 74–5
povidone-iodine solution 1
pretibial lacerations 37
proctoscopy, anal 81–2
prophylaxis, antibiotic 3–5

R
radiotherapy
   basal cell carcinoma 44
   keloid scar 43
recurrent varicose veins 53
retractor types 10–11

ring block anaesthesia 24–5
rodent ulcer 44–5

S
saphenous vein, long (vascular access) 28
scalpels 9–10
scar
   hypertrophic 42
   keloid 42–3
sclerotherapy (varicose veins) 53–6
scrubbing 1
sebaceous cyst 38–9
seborrheic wart 50
sedation, local anaesthesia 21
Seldinger technique, vascular access 28–9, 30
Seton procedure, anal procedures 95
shaving, skin 3
shock, treatment 27
sigmoidoscopy, anal 82–4
skin
   biopsy 49
   disinfecting 3
   lesions 35–50
skin graft, pinch 47–8
skin tag 37–8
   anal 87–8
solar keratosis 50
sphincterotomy (lateral/internal), anal procedures 90–2
squamous cell carcinoma 45
staples, wound 18
Steristrips 35, 37
subclavian vein access 29–31
subungual haematoma, nails 101–2
suprapubic catheterisation 116
surgeon's knot 18, 19
suture types 12–15

T
tag, skin 37–8
   anal 87–8
temporal artery biopsy 107–8
tissue glue 35, 36–7
toe amputation 108–9

total parenteral nutrition (TPN) 27, 32–3
tourniquet time 7
tourniquets 12
TPN *see* total parenteral nutrition
tunnelled venous lines 32–3

U
ulcers, venous 51
urethral catheterisation 110–15
urethral obstruction 116

V
varicose veins 51–67
  inversion stripping 64–5
  phlebectomies 65–7
  recurrent 53
vasectomy 120–2
veins, varicose 51–67
veins, vascular access
  internal jugular 31–2
  long saphenous 28
  subclavian 29–31
venous ulcers 51
verrucas 48–9

W
warts
  anal 95–7
  seborrheic 50
  viral 48–9
wedge excision, nails 102–4
wound
  clips 18–19
  infection 3–5
  staples 18
wounds, dirty 4, 36

Z
Zadek's operation (nails) 104–5

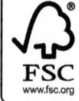

If you have any concerns about our products,
you can contact us on
ProductSafety@springernature.com

In case Publisher is established outside the EU,
the EU authorized representative is:
Springer Nature Customer Service Center GmbH
Europaplatz 3, 69115 Heidelberg, Germany

Printed by Libri Plureos GmbH
in Hamburg, Germany